Nutrition for Nursing
REVIEW MODULE EDITION 7.0

P9-DYY-739

Contributors

Honey C. Holman, MSN, RN

Debborah Williams, MSN, RN

Sheryl Sommer, PhD, RN, CNE

Janean Johnson, MSN, RN, CNE

Brenda S. Ball, MEd, BSN, RN

Peggy Leehy, MSN, RN

Consultants

Penny Fauber, PhD, MS, BSN, RN

Maria Sheilla Membrebe, MSN/Ed., RN, ONC, CMSRN, CBN

INTELLECTUAL PROPERTY NOTICE

ATI Nursing is a division of Assessment Technologies Institute®, LLC.

REPRINTED NOVEMBER 2021

Director of content review: Kristen Lawler

Director of development: Derek Prater

Project management: Tiffany Pavlik, Shannon Tierney

Coordination of content review: Honey C. Holman, Debborah Williams

Copy editing: Kelly Von Lunen, Bethany Phillips, Kya Rodgers

Layout: Spring Lenox, Maureen Bradshaw, Bethany Phillips

Illustrations: Randi Hardy

Online media: Brant Stacy, Ron Hanson, Britney Fuller, Barry Wilson

Cover design: Jason Buck

Interior book design: Spring Lenox

IMPORTANT NOTICE TO THE READER

User's Guide

Welcome to the Assessment Technologies Institute® Nutrition for Nursing Review Module Edition 7.0. The mission of ATI's Content Mastery Series® Review Modules is to provide user-friendly compendiums of nursing knowledge that will:
- Help you locate important information quickly.
- Assist in your learning efforts.
- Provide exercises for applying your nursing knowledge.
- Facilitate your entry into the nursing profession as a newly licensed nurse.

This newest edition of the Review Modules has been redesigned to optimize your learning experience. We've fit more content into less space and have done so in a way that will make it even easier for you to find and understand the information you need.

ORGANIZATION

This Review Module is organized into units covering principles of nutrition, clinical nutrition, and alterations in nutrition. Chapters within these units conform to one of two organizing principles for presenting the content.
- Nursing concepts
- Nutritional considerations for specific disorders

Nursing concepts chapters begin with an overview describing the central concept and its relevance to nursing. Subordinate themes are covered in outline form to demonstrate relationships and present the information in a clear, succinct manner.

Nutritional considerations for specific disorders chapters include an overview describing nutritional needs of clients who have the given disorder. These chapters cover assessments and data collection, nutritional guidelines, nursing interventions, and complications, if applicable.

ACTIVE LEARNING SCENARIOS AND APPLICATION EXERCISES

Each chapter includes opportunities for you to test your knowledge and to practice applying that knowledge. Active Learning Scenario exercises pose a nursing scenario and then direct you to use an ATI Active Learning Template (included at the back of this book) to record the important knowledge a nurse should apply to the scenario. An example is then provided to which you can compare your completed Active Learning Template. The Application Exercises include NCLEX-style questions, such as multiple-choice and multiple-select items, providing you with opportunities to practice answering the kinds of questions you might expect to see on ATI assessments or the NCLEX. After the Application Exercises, an answer key is provided, along with rationales.

NCLEX® CONNECTIONS

To prepare for the NCLEX, it is important to understand how the content in this Review Module is connected to the NCLEX test plan. You can find information on the detailed test plan at the National Council of State Boards of Nursing's website, www.ncsbn.org. When reviewing content in this Review Module, regularly ask yourself, "How does this content fit into the test plan, and what types of questions related to this content should I expect?"

To help you in this process, we've included NCLEX Connections at the beginning of each unit and with each question in the Application Exercises Answer Keys. The NCLEX Connections at the beginning of each unit point out areas of the detailed test plan that relate to the content within that unit. The NCLEX Connections attached to the Application Exercises Answer Keys demonstrate how each exercise fits within the detailed content outline.

These NCLEX Connections will help you understand how the detailed content outline is organized, starting with major client needs categories and subcategories and followed by related content areas and tasks. The major client needs categories are:
- Safe and Effective Care Environment
  - Management of Care
  - Safety and Infection Control
- Health Promotion and Maintenance
- Psychosocial Integrity
- Physiological Integrity
  - Basic Care and Comfort
  - Pharmacological and Parenteral Therapies
  - Reduction of Risk Potential
  - Physiological Adaptation

An NCLEX Connection might, for example, alert you that content within a unit is related to:
- Basic Care and Comfort
  - Nutrition and Oral Hydration
    - Manage the client who has an alteration in nutritional intake.

QSEN COMPETENCIES

As you use the Review Modules, you will note the integration of the Quality and Safety Education for Nurses (QSEN) competencies throughout the chapters. These competencies are integral components of the curriculum of many nursing programs in the United States and prepare you to provide safe, high-quality care as a newly licensed nurse. Icons appear to draw your attention to the six QSEN competencies.

Safety: The minimization of risk factors that could cause injury or harm while promoting quality care and maintaining a secure environment for clients, self, and others.

Patient-Centered Care: The provision of caring and compassionate, culturally sensitive care that addresses clients' physiological, psychological, sociological, spiritual, and cultural needs, preferences, and values.

Evidence-Based Practice: The use of current knowledge from research and other credible sources, on which to base clinical judgment and client care.

Informatics: The use of information technology as a communication and information-gathering tool that supports clinical decision-making and scientifically based nursing practice.

Quality Improvement: Care related and organizational processes that involve the development and implementation of a plan to improve health care services and better meet clients' needs.

Teamwork and Collaboration: The delivery of client care in partnership with multidisciplinary members of the health care team to achieve continuity of care and positive client outcomes.

ICONS

Icons are used throughout the Review Module to draw your attention to particular areas. Keep an eye out for these icons.

(N) This icon is used for NCLEX Connections.

(G) This icon indicates gerontological considerations, or knowledge specific to the care of older adult clients.

Qs This icon is used for content related to safety and is a QSEN competency. When you see this icon, take note of safety concerns or steps that nurses can take to ensure client safety and a safe environment.

QPCC This icon is a QSEN competency that indicates the importance of a holistic approach to providing care.

QEBP This icon, a QSEN competency, points out the integration of research into clinical practice.

QI This icon is a QSEN competency and highlights the use of information technology to support nursing practice.

QQI This icon is used to focus on the QSEN competency of integrating planning processes to meet clients' needs.

QTC This icon highlights the QSEN competency of care delivery using an interprofessional approach.

M◇ This icon appears at the top-right of pages and indicates availability of an online media supplement, such as a graphic, animation, or video. If you have an electronic copy of the Review Module, this icon will appear alongside clickable links to media supplements. If you have a hard copy version of the Review Module, visit www.atitesting.com for details on how to access these features.

FEEDBACK

ATI welcomes feedback regarding this Review Module. Please provide comments to comments@atitesting.com.

As needed updates to the Review Modules are identified, changes to the text are made for subsequent printings of the book and for subsequent releases of the electronic version. For the printed books, print runs are based on when existing stock is depleted. For the electronic versions, a number of factors influence the update schedule. As such, ATI encourages faculty and students to refer to the Review Module addendums for information on what updates have been made. These addendums—which are available in the Help/FAQs on the student site and the Resources/eBooks & Active Learning on the faculty site— are updated regularly and always include the most current information on updates to the Review Modules.

Table of Contents

When reviewing the following chapters, keep in mind the relevant topics and tasks of the NCLEX outline, in particular:

Health Promotion and Maintenance

AGING PROCESS
Provide care and education for the newborn, infant, and toddler client from birth through 2 years.

Provide care and education for the adult client ages 65 years and over.

ANTE/INTRA/POSTPARTUM AND NEWBORN CARE: Provide prenatal care and education.

HEALTH PROMOTION/DISEASE PREVENTION: Educate the client on actions to promote/maintain health and prevent disease.

HEALTH SCREENING: Perform targeted screening assessments.

Basic Care and Comfort

NUTRITION AND ORAL HYDRATION
Consider client choices regarding meeting nutritional requirements and/or maintaining dietary restrictions, including mention of specific food items.

Initiate calorie counts for clients.

Apply knowledge of mathematics to client nutrition.

Physiological Adaptation

FLUID AND ELECTROLYTE IMBALANCES: Manage the care of the client with a fluid and electrolyte imbalance.

UNIT 1   PRINCIPLES OF NUTRITION

CHAPTER 1   *Sources of Nutrition*

Nutrients absorbed in the diet determine, to a large degree, the health of the body. Deficiencies or excesses can contribute to a poor state of health. Essential nutrients are those that the body cannot manufacture, and the absence of essential nutrients can cause deficiency diseases.

Components of nutritive sources are carbohydrates and fiber, protein, lipids (fats), vitamins, minerals and electrolytes, and water. Carbohydrates, fats, and proteins are all energy-yielding nutrients. A healthy eating pattern includes foods that provide all essential nutrients, and allows a broad assortment of food sources.

DIETARY REFERENCE INTAKES

Dietary Reference Intakes (DRIs) are developed by the Institute of Medicine's Standing Committee on the Scientific Evaluation of Dietary Reference Intakes.

- DRIs are useful in understanding the food intake patterns of large groups, planning nutrition program standards (Supplemental Nutrition Assistance program [SNAP]), and helping individuals.
- DRIs are comprised of the following reference values.
  - Recommended Dietary Allowances (RDAs): The amount of a particular nutrient that most healthy people in a similar life-stage and sex will need to decrease the risk of chronic disease.
  - Estimated Average Requirement (EAR): The amount of a nutrient required to meet basic requirements for half of the people in a particular population. This reference is often used by researchers and policy makers, and is used to help determine RDAs.
  - Adequate Intake (AI): The amount of a nutrient that most people in a group or population consume. This is helpful when there is not enough data to establish an RDA for a nutrient.
  - Tolerable Upper Intake Level (UL): The upper limit on the amount of a particular nutrient, or the maximum an individual should consume. ULs are used when a nutrient is known to have adverse effects.
  - Acceptable Macronutrient Distribution Ranges (AMDRs): The recommended percentages of intake for energy-yielding nutrients (carbohydrates, fat, protein).
- Clients can use DRIs as a guide for nutrition intake, but should also consider individual factors that increase nutrient needs (disease, injury).

Carbohydrates and fiber

All carbohydrates are organic compounds composed of carbon, hydrogen, and oxygen (CHO). The main function of carbohydrates is to provide energy for the body.

- The average minimum amount (DRI) of carbohydrates needed to fuel the brain is 130 g/day for adults and children. Median carbohydrate intake is 305 g/day for males aged 20 years and older, and 228 g/day for adults, children, and females in the same age range. The AMDR for carbohydrates is 45% to 65% of calories.
- Carbohydrates provide energy for cellular work, and help to regulate protein and fat metabolism. Adequate amounts of protein in the diet creates a protein-sparing effect, which results in protein being spared from energy use to perform its other essential functions. Brain and nervous system tissue require carbohydrates for maximum effective functioning.

TYPES OF CARBOHYDRATES (1.1)

Carbohydrates are classified according to the number of saccharide units making up their structure.

Monosaccharides: simple carbohydrates (glucose, fructose, and galactose)
Disaccharides: simple carbohydrates (sucrose, lactose, and maltose)
Polysaccharides: complex carbohydrates (starch, fiber, and glycogen)

CONSIDERATIONS

- The liver converts fructose and galactose into glucose, which is then released in the bloodstream. This elevates blood glucose levels, which causes the release of insulin from the pancreas. With insulin production, glucose is moved out of the bloodstream into cells in order to meet energy needs.
- The body digests 95% of starch within 1 to 4 hr after ingestion. Digestion occurs mainly in the small intestine using pancreatic amylase to reduce complex carbohydrates into disaccharides.
- Glycogen is the stored carbohydrate energy source found in the liver and muscles. It is a vital source of backup energy, but is only available in limited supply.
- To maintain glucose levels between meals, glucose is released through the breakdown of liver glycogen.
- Digestible carbohydrates provide 4 cal/g of energy and make blood glucose levels more stable.

1.1 Carbohydrates at a glance

	EXAMPLE (SOURCES)	FUNCTION
Monosaccharides	Glucose (corn syrup), fructose (fruits), galactose (found in milk)	Basic energy for cells
Disaccharides	Sucrose (table sugar), lactose (milk sugar), maltose (malt sugar)	Energy, aids calcium and phosphorus absorption (lactose)
Polysaccharides	Starches (grains, legumes, root vegetables), fiber (whole grains, fruits, vegetables)	Energy storage (starches), digestive aid (fiber)

FIBER

Fiber is categorized as a carbohydrate.
- Dietary fiber is the substance in plant foods that is indigestible. Types are pectin, gum, cellulose, and oligosaccharides.
- Fiber is important for proper bowel elimination. It adds bulk to the feces and stimulates peristalsis to ease elimination.
- Fiber helps to lower cholesterol and lessen the incidence of intestinal cancers. It has also been shown to help keep blood glucose levels stable by slowing the rate of glucose absorption.
- Total fiber AI is 25 g/day for females and 38 g/day for males.
- The fermentation and metabolization of fiber in the colon provides 1.5 to 2.5 cal/g of energy, depending on the type.

Proteins

Proteins are provided by plant and animal sources. They are formed by linking amino acids in various combinations for specific use by the body.

TYPES OF PROTEINS

There are two types of proteins. Each is obtained from the diet in various ways.

Complete proteins, from animal sources and soy, contain sufficient amounts of all nine essential amino acids.

Incomplete proteins, generally from plant sources, can contain an insufficient number or quantity of amino acids, which limits the ability for protein synthesis.
- Complementary proteins are incomplete proteins that, when combined, provide a complete protein. It is not necessary to consume complementary proteins at the same time to form a complete protein; instead, consuming a variety of complementary proteins over the course of the day is sufficient.
- Examples of incomplete protein pairs that provide complete protein include black beans with rice and hummus with crackers.

CONSIDERATIONS

- Proteins have many metabolic functions.
  - Tissue-building and maintenance
  - Balance of nitrogen and water
  - Backup energy
  - Support of metabolic processes
    - Nitrogen balance
    - Transportation of nutrients, other vital substances
  - Support of the immune system
  - Facilitating acid-base, fluid, and electrolyte balance
  - Formation of neurotransmitters, enzymes antibodies, peptide hormones, breast milk, mucus, histamine, and sperm
- Three main factors influence the body's requirement for protein.
  - Tissue growth needs
  - Quality of the dietary protein
  - Added needs due to illness

- The RDA of protein is 0.8 g/kg for healthy adults. Protein's acceptable macronutrient distribution range (AMDR) for adults is 10% to 35% of total calories.
- Underconsumption can lead to protein energy malnutrition (PEM). Kwashiorkor and marasmus are two disorders caused by extreme PEM. These serious disorders are caused by a lack of protein ingestion.
- Protein provides 4 cal/g of energy.

Lipids

- The chemical group of fats is called lipids, and they are available from many sources.
  - Dark meat
  - Poultry skin
  - Dairy foods
  - Added oils (margarine, butter, shortening, oils, lard)
- Fat is an essential nutrient for the body. It serves as a concentrated form of stored energy for the body and supplies important tissue needs.
  - Hormone production
  - Structural material for cell walls
  - Protective padding for vital organs
  - Insulation to maintain body temperature
  - Covering for nerve fibers
  - Aid in the absorption of fat-soluble vitamins

TYPES OF FATS

Fats are divided into three categories: triglycerides, phospholipids, and sterols. Triglycerides are further comprised of fatty acids, which include saturated fatty acids and unsaturated fatty acids.

Triglycerides

Triglycerides total 95% of fat in food. They combine with glycerol to supply energy to the body, allow fat-soluble vitamin transport, and form adipose tissue that protects internal organs.
- **Saturated fatty acids** are solid at room temperature, and are found primarily in animal sources.
- **Unsaturated fatty acids**, including monounsaturated and polyunsaturated fatty acids, are usually from plant sources and help reduce health risks.
  - Sources of **monounsaturated fatty acids** include olives, canola oil, avocado, peanuts, and other nuts.
  - Sources of **polyunsaturated fatty acids** include corn, wheat germ, soybean, safflower, sunflower, and fish.
- **Essential fatty acids**, made from broken down fats, must be supplied by the diet. Essential fatty acids, including omega-3 and omega-6, are used to support blood clotting, blood pressure, inflammatory responses, and many other metabolic processes.

Phospholipids

Phospholipids (e.g., lecithin) are important to cell membrane structure, as well as the transport of fat-soluble substances across the cell membrane.

Sterols

Sterols (e.g., cholesterol) are found in the tissues of animals, and are not an essential nutrient because the liver is able to produce enough to meet needs.

If cholesterol is consumed in excess, it can build up in the tissues, causing congestion and increasing the risk for cardiovascular disease.

CONSIDERATIONS

- The AMDR for fats is approximately 20% to 35% of total calories. 10% or less of total calories should come from saturated fat sources.
- A low intake of dietary cholesterol is associated with reduced risks of cardiovascular disease (CVD) and obesity.
- A diet high in fat is linked to CVD, hypertension, and diabetes mellitus.
  - The exception is for children under 2 years of age, who need a higher amount of fat to form brain tissue.
  - Conversely, a diet with less than 10% of fat cannot supply adequate amounts of essential fatty acids and results in a cachectic (wasting) state.
- The majority of lipid metabolism occurs after fat reaches the small intestine, where the gallbladder secretes concentrated bile, which acts as an emulsifier and enables the breakdown of fat down into smaller particles for digestion. At the same time, the pancreas secretes pancreatic lipase, which breaks down fat. Intestinal cells absorb the majority of the end products of digestion, with some being excreted in the feces.
  - **Very-low-density lipoproteins (VLDL)** carry triglycerides to the cells.
  - **Low-density lipoproteins (LDL)** carry cholesterol to the tissue cells.
  - **High-density lipoproteins (HDL)** remove excess cholesterol from the cells, and transport it to the liver for disposal.
- Lipids provide 9 cal/g of energy and are the densest form of stored energy.

Vitamins

Vitamins are organic substances required for many enzymatic reactions. The main function of vitamins is to be a catalyst for metabolic functions and chemical reactions.
- There are 13 essential vitamins, each having a specialized function.
- There are two classes of vitamins.
  - **Water-soluble:** Vitamins C and B-complex
  - **Fat-soluble:** Vitamins A, D, E, and K
- Vitamins yield no usable energy for the body, but they are needed for energy to be metabolized.

WATER-SOLUBLE VITAMINS

Vitamin C

Vitamin C (ascorbic acid) aids in tissue building and metabolic reactions (healing, collagen formation, iron absorption, immune system function).
- Vitamin C is found in citrus fruits (oranges, lemons), tomatoes, peppers, green leafy vegetables, and strawberries.
- Stress and illness, as well as cigarette smoking, increases the need for vitamin C. Cigarette smokers are advised to increase Vitamin C intake by 35 mg/day due to increased oxidative stress and metabolic turnover.
- Severe deficiency causes scurvy, a hemorrhagic disease with diffuse tissue bleeding, painful limbs/joints, weak bones, and swollen gums/loose teeth. While scurvy can be fatal, it can also be cured with moderate doses of vitamin C for several days.

B-complex vitamins

B-complex vitamins have many functions in cell metabolism. Each one has a varied duty. Many partner with other B vitamins for metabolic reactions. Most affect energy, metabolism, and neurologic function. Sources for B vitamins almost always include green leafy vegetables and unprocessed or enriched grains.

Thiamin (B_1) functions as a coenzyme in energy metabolism, promotes appetite, and assists with muscle actions through its role in nerve functioning.
- Deficiency results in beriberi (ataxia, confusion, anorexia, tachycardia), headache, weight loss, and fatigue.
- Food sources are widespread in almost all plant and animal tissues, especially meats, grains, and legumes.

Riboflavin (B_2) works as a coenzyme to release energy from cells.
- Deficiency results in cheilosis (manifestations include scales and cracks on lips and in corners of the mouth), smooth/swollen red tongue (also called glossitis), and dermatitis of the ears, nose, and mouth.
- Dietary sources include milk, meats, and dark leafy vegetables.

Niacin (B_3) aids in the metabolism of fats, glucose, and alcohol, and synthesis of steroid hormones, cholesterol, and fatty acids.
- Deficiency causes pellagra (manifestations include sun-sensitive skin lesions, and gastrointestinal issues with impaired food digestion and excretion, as well as nutrient absorption and neurologic findings [anxiety, insomnia, confusion, paranoia]).
- Sources include meats, legumes, milk, whole grain and enriched breads and cereals.

Pyridoxine/Vitamin B_6 is needed for cellular function and synthesis of hemoglobin, neurotransmitters, and niacin.
- Deficiency causes macrocytic anemia and CNS disturbances.
- High intake of supplements can cause sensory neuropathy.
- Widespread food sources include meats, grains, and legumes.

Pantothenic acid is involved in the metabolism of carbohydrates, fats, and proteins as part of coenzyme A.
- Deficiency is extremely rare, but results in generalized body system failure.
- Rich sources include meats, whole grain cereals, dried peas and beans.

Biotin serves as a coenzyme used in fatty acid synthesis, amino acid metabolism, and the formation of glucose.
- Deficiency is rare, but results in neurologic findings (depression, fatigue), hair loss, and scaly red rash.
- Widespread food sources include eggs, milk, and dark green vegetables.

Folate is required for hemoglobin and amino acid synthesis, new cell synthesis, and prevention of neural tube defects in utero. (Folic acid is the synthetic form.)
- Deficiency causes megaloblastic anemia, CNS disturbances, and fetal neural tube defects (spina bifida, anencephaly). It is important that all clients of child-bearing age get an adequate amount of folate due to neural tube formation occurring early in gestation, often before a client knows they are pregnant. Q EBP
- Folate occurs naturally in a variety of foods including liver, dark-green leafy vegetables, orange juice, and legumes.

Cobalamin (B₁₂) is necessary for folate activation and red blood cell maturation.
- Deficiency causes pernicious anemia and is seen mostly in clients who follow a strict vegan diet (B₁₂ is found solely in foods of animal origin), and those who have an absence of intrinsic factor needed for absorption of B₁₂.
- Sources include meat, shellfish, eggs, and dairy products.

FAT-SOLUBLE VITAMINS

- All fat-soluble vitamins have the possibility for toxicity due to their ability to be stored in the body for long periods of time.
- Absorption of fat-soluble vitamins is dependent on the body's ability to absorb dietary fat. Fat digestion can be interrupted by any number of conditions, particularly those that affect the secretion of fat-converting enzymes, and conditions of the small intestine. Clients who have cystic fibrosis, celiac disease, Crohn's disease, or intestinal bypasses are at risk for deficiencies.
- Clients who have liver disease should be careful not to take more than the daily recommendations of fat-soluble vitamins, as excess is stored in the liver and adipose tissue.

Vitamin A

Vitamin A (retinol, beta-carotene) contributes to vision health, tissue strength and growth, and embryonic development. Retinoids are found in animal foods and are the active form of vitamin A. Carotenoids are found in plants and are a precursor form of vitamin A, which the body converts to the usable form as needed.
- Care should be taken when administered to pregnant clients as some forms have teratogenic effects on the fetus.
- Deficiency results in vision changes, xerophthalmia (dryness and hardening of the cornea), GI disturbances, and hyperkeratosis.
- Food sources include fatty fish, egg yolks, butter, cream, and dark yellow/orange fruits and vegetables (carrots, yams, apricots, squash, cantaloupe).
- Toxicity can result from retinoids, and is more common in clients who are taking vitamin A supplements.

1.2 Water-soluble vitamins at a glance

	MAJOR ACTIONS	MAJOR SOURCES	DEFICIENCY
Vitamin C (ascorbic acid)	Antioxidant, tissue building, iron absorption	Citrus fruits and juices, vegetables	Scurvy, decreased iron absorption, bleeding gums
Thiamin (B₁)	Muscle energy, energy metabolism	Meats, grains, legumes	Beriberi, headache, weight loss, fatigue
Riboflavin (B₂)	Assists with releasing energy from cells	Milk, meats, dark leafy vegetables	Skin eruptions, cracked lips, red swollen tongue
Niacin (B₃)	Metabolism of fat, glucose, and alcohol; synthesis of fatty acids, cholesterol, and steroid hormones	Liver, nuts, legumes	Pellagra, skin lesions, GI and CNS findings, dementia
Pantothenic acid	Carbohydrate, fat, and protein metabolism	Meats, whole grain cereals, dried peas and beans.	Rare; Generalized body system failure
Pyridoxine (B₆)	Cellular function, heme and neurotransmitter synthesis	Meats, grains, and legumes	Macrocytic anemia, CNS disturbances, poor growth
Folate	Synthesis of amino acids and hemoglobin, formation of fetal neural tube	Liver, green leafy vegetables, legumes	Megaloblastic anemia, CNS disturbance
Cobalamin (B₁₂)	Folate activation, red blood cell maturation	Meats, clams, oysters, eggs, dairy products	Pernicious anemia, GI findings, poor muscle coordination, paresthesia of the hands and feet
Biotin	Fatty acid synthesis, amino acid metabolism, glucose formation	Eggs, milk, dark green vegetables	Rare; scaly rash, hair loss, depression, fatigue

1.3 Fat-soluble vitamins at a glance

	MAJOR ACTIONS	MAJOR SOURCES	DEFICIENCY
Vitamin A	Normal vision, tissue strength, growth and immune system function	Orange/yellow fruits and vegetables, fatty fish, dairy	Reduced night vision, dry/thick corneas, mucosa changes
Vitamin D	Maintain blood calcium and phosphorus, aid in bone development	Fish, fortified dairy products, egg yolks, sunlight	Low blood calcium, fragile bones, rickets, osteomalacia in adults
Vitamin E	Protects vitamin A from oxidation	Vegetable oils, grains, nuts, dark green vegetables	Anemia, edema and skin lesions in infants
Vitamin K	Essential for prothrombin synthesis, aids in bone metabolism	Green leafy vegetables, eggs	Increased bleeding times

Vitamin D

Vitamin D assists in the absorption of calcium and phosphorus, and aids in bone mineralization.
- Sunlight enables the body to synthesize vitamin D in the skin.
- Deficiency results in bone demineralization, and extreme deficiency can cause rickets and osteomalacia. Excess consumption can cause hypercalcemia.
- Food sources include fatty fish, eggs, and fortified products (ready-to-eat cereals, milk, orange juice).

Vitamin E

Vitamin E is an antioxidant that helps to preserve lung and red blood cell membranes.
- Deficiency rare, but results in anemia and can cause edema and skin lesions in infants.
- Food sources include vegetable oils and certain nuts.

Vitamin K

Vitamin K assists in blood clotting and bone maintenance.
- Deficiency results in increased bleeding time.
- Used as an antidote for excess anticoagulants (warfarin).
- Vitamin K is found in carrots, eggs, and dark green vegetables (spinach, broccoli, asparagus).

Minerals and electrolytes

Minerals are inorganic elements, are available in an abundance of food sources, and are used at every cellular level for metabolic exchanges. Minerals are divided into major and trace.

Electrolytes are electrically-charged minerals that cause physiological reactions that maintain homeostasis. Major electrolytes include sodium, potassium, and chloride.

MAJOR MINERALS

Major minerals occur in larger amounts (more than 5 g) in the body, and 100 mg or more is required through dietary sources each day. The seven major minerals are calcium, phosphorus, sodium, potassium, magnesium, chloride, and sulfur.

Sodium (Na)

MAJOR ACTIONS: Maintains fluid volume, allows muscle contractions, contributes to nerve impulses

MAJOR SOURCES: Table salt, added salts, processed foods

FINDINGS OF DEFICIENCY: Muscle cramping, memory loss, anorexia

FINDINGS OF EXCESS: Fluid retention, hypertension, disorientation

NURSING ACTIONS: Monitor level of consciousness, edema, and blood pressure.

Potassium (K)

MAJOR ACTIONS: Maintains fluid volume inside cells, muscle action

MAJOR SOURCES: Oranges, dried fruits, tomatoes, avocados, dried peas, meats, broccoli, bananas, dairy products, meats, whole grains, potato

FINDINGS OF DEFICIENCY: Dysrhythmias, muscle cramps, confusion

FINDINGS OF EXCESS: Dysrhythmia, muscle weakness, irritability, confusion, numbness in extremities

NURSING ACTIONS: Monitor cardiac status and ECG. Give oral preparations (tabs, elixirs) with meals to minimize GI irritation.

Chloride (Cl)

MAJOR ACTIONS: Assists with intracellular and extracellular fluid balance, and aids acid–based balance and digestion

MAJOR SOURCES: Table salt, added salts, processed foods

FINDINGS OF DEFICIENCY: Rare; muscle cramps, anorexia

FINDINGS OF EXCESS: Vomiting

NURSING ACTIONS: Monitor sodium levels.

Calcium (Ca)

MAJOR ACTIONS: Bones/teeth formation, blood pressure, blood clotting, nerve transmission

MAJOR SOURCES: Dairy, broccoli, kale, fortified grains

FINDINGS OF DEFICIENCY: Tetany, positive Chvostek's and Trousseau's signs, ECG changes, osteoporosis in adults, poor growth in children

FINDINGS OF EXCESS: Constipation, renal stones, lethargy, depressed deep-tendon reflexes

NURSING ACTIONS: Monitor ECG and respiratory status. Give PO tabs with vitamin D.

Magnesium (Mg)

MAJOR ACTIONS: Bone formation, catalyst for many enzyme reactions, nerve/muscle function, smooth muscle relaxation

MAJOR SOURCES: Green leafy vegetables, nuts, whole grains, tuna, halibut, chocolate

FINDINGS OF DEFICIENCY: Weakness, dysrhythmias, convulsions, increased blood pressure, anorexia

FINDINGS OF EXCESS: Diarrhea, nausea, muscle weakness, hypotension, bradycardia, lethargy

NURSING ACTIONS: Follow seizure precautions, and monitor level of consciousness and vital signs. Qs

Phosphorus (P)

MAJOR ACTIONS: Energy transfer of RNA/DNA, acid–base balance, bone and teeth formation

MAJOR SOURCES: Dairy, peas, meat, eggs, legumes

FINDINGS OF DEFICIENCY: Unknown

FINDINGS OF EXCESS: Decreased blood calcium levels

NURSING ACTIONS: Evaluate the use of antacids (note type) and the use of alcohol (alcohol impairs absorption).

Sulfur (S)

MAJOR ACTIONS: A component of vitamin structure, by-product of protein metabolism

MAJOR SOURCES: Proteins

FINDINGS OF DEFICIENCY: Only seen in severe protein malnourishment

FINDINGS OF EXCESS: Toxicity does not result in any health issues

NURSING ACTIONS: Sulfur levels are not usually monitored.

TRACE MINERALS

Trace minerals, also called micronutrients, are required by the body in amounts of less than 5 g, and 20 mg or less is required through dietary sources each day. The nine trace elements are iron, iodine, zinc, copper, manganese, chromium, selenium, molybdenum, and fluoride.

Iodine

Iodine is used for synthesis of thyroxine, the thyroid hormone that helps regulate metabolism. Iodine is taken up by the thyroid. When iodine is lacking, the thyroid gland enlarges, creating a goiter. Too much iodine can result in thyrotoxicosis.

- Grown food sources vary widely and are dependent on the iodine content of the soil in which they were grown.
- Seafood provides a good amount of iodine. Table salt in the U.S. is fortified with iodine, so deficiencies are not as prevalent.
- The RDA is 150 mcg for adults.

Iron

Iron is responsible for oxygen distribution to hemoglobin and myoglobin.

- The body recycles unused iron from dying red blood cells and stores it for later use.
- Iron in food consists of two forms: heme iron found in meat, fish, and poultry and non-heme iron found in grains, legumes, and vegetables.
- Iron supplements can cause constipation, nausea, vomiting, diarrhea, and teeth discoloration (liquid form). They can be taken with food to avert gastrointestinal manifestations, and nurses should encourage fresh fruits, vegetables, and a high-fiber diet.
- Supplements that are unneeded can become toxic.
- Vitamin C increases the absorption of iron.
- Clients during the menstruating years, older infants and toddlers, and pregnant clients are at risk for iron deficiency anemia.
- Toxicity can occur when there is too much iron stored in the body.

Fluoride

Fluoride forms a bond with calcium and thus accumulates in calcified body tissue (bones and teeth). Water with added fluoride protects against dental cavities.

- Deficiency can result in dental caries, and increase the risk for osteoporosis.
- Toxicity can result in fluorosis, itching, and chest pain.

Water

Water is the most basic of nutrients. The body can maintain itself for several weeks on its food stores of energy, but it cannot survive without water/hydration for more than a few days. Water makes up the largest portion of our total body weight and is crucial for all fluid and cellular functions.

- Fluid balance is essential for optimum health and bodily function.
- The balance of fluid is a dynamic process regulated by the release of hormones.
- Water leaves the body via the kidneys, skin, lungs, and feces. The greatest elimination is through the kidneys. Other loss factors include bleeding, vomiting, and rapid respirations.
- To maintain a balance between intake and output, intake should approximate output. Healthy adults lose approximately 1000 mL of water daily through insensible losses (respirations, skin, fecal), and to get rid of metabolic wastes needs to excrete at least 500 mL of urine daily. Therefore, the minimum daily amount of water intake needed is 1,500 mL.
- Most water intake is from drinking fluids; water is also present in solid sources (lettuce, gelatin, soup, melons). Under normal conditions, the AI for adult water intake for females is 2.7 L/day, of which 2.2 L should be from fluids; and for males 3.7 L/day, of which 3 L should be from fluids. Ⓠᴇʙᴘ
- Additional hydration can be required for athletes, persons with fever/illness (vomiting, diarrhea), and those in hot climate conditions. Fluid replacement can occur orally, enterally, or IV.
- Young children and older adults dehydrate more rapidly.
- Assessment for proper hydration should include skin turgor, mental status, orthostatic blood pressures, urine output and concentration, and moistness of mucous membranes
- Thirst is a late indicator of the need for hydration, especially in older adults. Ⓖ
- Some individuals can have an aversion to drinking water, and should be encouraged to explore other options (fresh fruits, fruit juices, flavored gelatin, frozen treats, soups).
- Caffeinated drinks have a mild diuretic effect. However, tolerance develops in clients who regularly consume caffeinated beverages, which results in little to no effect on fluid volume.

Phytonutrients

Also called phytochemicals, phytonutrients occur naturally in plants. They can have positive health effects (detoxifying the body, stimulating the immune system, promoting hormone balance, serving as antioxidants).

- They are found in fruits, vegetables, green tea, legumes, whole grains, and broccoli.
- No recommendations for intake of phytonutrients exists at this time.

Application Exercises

1. A nurse is educating a client who has anemia about dietary intake of iron. Which of the following is a non-heme source of iron?
   A. Ground beef
   B. Dried beans
   C. Salmon
   D. Turkey

2. A nurse is discussing foods that are high in vitamin D with a client who is unable to be out in the sunlight. Which of the following should be included in the teaching?
   A. 1 cup steamed long-grain brown rice
   B. 6 medium raw strawberries
   C. ½ cup boiled Brussels sprouts
   D. 2 large, poached eggs

3. A nurse is reviewing dietary recommendations with a group of clients at a health fair. Which of the following information should the nurse include?
   A. "Fats should be 5% to 15% of daily calorie intake."
   B. "Make protein 10% to 35% of total calories each day."
   C. "Consume 1,500 mL of water from liquids and solids daily."
   D. "The body needs 40 mg of iron each day."

4. A nurse is conducting a nutritional class on minerals and electrolytes. The nurse should include which of the following foods is a major source of magnesium?
   A. Tuna
   B. Tomatoes
   C. Eggs
   D. Oranges

5. A nurse is discussing health problems associated with nutrient deficiencies with a group of clients. Which of the following conditions is associated with a deficiency of vitamin C? (Select all that apply.)
   A. Dysrhythmias
   B. Scurvy
   C. Pernicious anemia
   D. Megaloblastic anemia
   E. Bleeding gums

Active Learning Scenario

A school nurse is conducting a nutritional class for a group of athletes. Use the ATI Active Learning Template: Basic Concept to complete this item.

RELATED CONTENT
- Describe two types of protein.
- Describe complimentary proteins.
- Describe three main factors influencing the body's requirement for protein.

Application Exercises Key

1. A. Ground beef is an animal product, which provides heme iron.
   B. **CORRECT:** Dried beans provide non-heme iron, as do other legumes, vegetables, and grains.
   C. Salmon is an animal product, which provides heme iron.
   D. Turkey is an animal product, which provides heme iron.

   Ⓝ *NCLEX® Connection: Basic Care and Comfort, Nutrition and Oral Hydration*

2. A. Long-grain brown rice does not contain vitamin D.
   B. Strawberries do not contain vitamin D.
   C. Brussels sprouts do not contain vitamin D.
   D. **CORRECT:** Include eggs as a food that is high in vitamin D.

   Ⓝ *NCLEX® Connection: Basic Care and Comfort, Nutrition and Oral Hydration*

3. A. Fats should be 20% to 35% of daily calorie intake.
   B. **CORRECT:** The recommendation for protein intake is 10% to 35% of total daily calories.
   C. Recommended water intake from liquids or solids is 2.7 L/day for females and 3.7 L/day for males.
   D. Iron is a trace mineral, which means the body needs 20 mg or less daily.

   Ⓝ *NCLEX® Connection: Basic Care and Comfort, Nutrition and Oral Hydration*

4. A. **CORRECT:** Tuna and halibut are major sources of magnesium.
   B. Green, leafy vegetables are a good source of magnesium.
   C. Nuts are a major source of magnesium.
   D. Chocolate is a major source of magnesium.

   Ⓝ *NCLEX® Connection: Physiological Adaptation, Fluid and Electrolyte Imbalances*

5. A. Dysrhythmias are associated with a potassium deficiency.
   B. **CORRECT:** Scurvy is associated with a vitamin C deficiency.
   C. Pernicious anemia is associated a deficiency of vitamin B_{12}.
   D. Megaloblastic anemia is associated with a deficiency of folate.
   E. **CORRECT:** Bleeding gums is a condition that results from vitamin C deficiency.

   Ⓝ *NCLEX® Connection: Physiological Adaptation, Illness Management*

Active Learning Scenario Key

Using the ATI Active Learning Template: Basic Concept

RELATED CONTENT

- Types of protein
  - Complete proteins, from animal sources and soy, contain sufficient amounts of all nine essential amino acids.
  - Incomplete proteins, generally from plant sources, can contain an insufficient number or quantify of amino acids, which limits the ability for protein synthesis.
- Complementary proteins
  - Complementary proteins are those food sources that are incomplete proteins eaten alone, but together are equivalent to a complete protein. It is not necessary to consume complementary proteins at the same time to form a complete protein; instead, consuming a variety of complementary proteins over the course of the day is sufficient.
- Main factors influencing the body's requirement for protein
  - Tissue growth needs
  - Quality of the dietary protein
  - Added needs due to illness

Ⓝ *NCLEX® Connection: Health Promotion and Maintenance, Health Promotion/Disease Prevention*

UNIT 1   PRINCIPLES OF NUTRITION

CHAPTER 2   *Ingestion, Digestion, Absorption, and Metabolism*

Ingestion is the process of consuming food by the mouth, and moving it through the digestive system. Digestion is a systemic process that includes the breakdown and absorption of nutrients.

Absorption occurs as components of nutrients pass through the digestive system into the bloodstream and lymphatic system.

Metabolism is the sum of all chemical processes that occur on a cellular level to maintain homeostasis. Metabolism is comprised of catabolism (the breaking down of substances with the resultant release of energy) and anabolism (the use of energy to build or repair substances).

Energy nutrients are metabolized to provide carbon dioxide, water, and adenosine triphosphate (ATP). Excess energy nutrients are stored; glucose is converted to glycogen and stored in the liver and muscle tissue; surplus glucose is converted to fat; glycerol and fatty acids are reassembled into triglycerides and stored in adipose tissue; and amino acids make body proteins. The liver removes nitrogen from amino acids, and the remaining product is converted to glucose or fat for energy. Body cells first use available ATP for growth and repair, then use glycogen and stored fat.

METABOLIC RATE

Metabolic rate refers to the speed at which food energy is burned.

- **Basal metabolic rate (BMR)**, also called basal energy expenditure (BEE), refers to the amount of energy used in 24 hr for involuntary activities of the body (maintaining body temperature, heartbeat, circulation, and respirations). This rate is determined while at rest, and following a 12-hr fast.
- **Resting metabolic rate (RMR)**, also called resting energy expenditure (REE), refers to the calories needed for involuntary activities of the body at rest. This rate does not consider the 12-hr fast criteria.
- BMR is affected by lean body mass and hormones. Body surface area, age, and sex are also factors that contribute to BMR.
- In general, males have a higher metabolic rate than females due to their higher amount of body muscle and decreased amount of fat.
- Thyroid function tests can be used as an indirect measure of BMR.
- Acute stress causes an increase in metabolism, blood glucose levels, and protein catabolism.
  - A major nutritional concern during acute stress is protein deficiency as stress hormones break down protein at a very rapid rate.
  - Protein deficiency increases the risk of complications from severe trauma or critical illness (skin breakdown, delayed wound healing, infections, organ failure, ulcers, impaired medication tolerance).
  - Protein requirements can be increased to more than 2 g/kg of body weight, or up to 25% of total calories, depending on the client's age and prior nutritional status. ⓠEBP
- Any catabolic illness (surgery, extensive burns) increases the body's requirement for calories to meet the demands of an increased BMR.
- Disease and sepsis also increase metabolic demands and can lead to starvation/death.

FACTORS AFFECTING METABOLIC RATE

INCREASE BMR
- Lean, muscular body build
- Exposure to extreme temperatures
- Prolonged stress
- Rapid growth periods (infancy, puberty)
- Pregnancy

Lactation
- Physical conditioning

DECREASE BMR
- Short, overweight body build
- Starvation/malnutrition
- Age-related loss of lean body masses

Conditions

INCREASE METABOLISM
- Fever
- Involuntary muscle tremors (shivering, Parkinson's)
- Hyperthyroidism
- Cancer
- Cardiac failure
- Burns
- Surgery/wound healing
- HIV/AIDS

DECREASE METABOLISM: Hypothyroidism

Medications

INCREASE BMR
- Epinephrine
- Levothyroxine
- Ephedrine sulfate

DECREASE BMR
- Opioids
- Muscle relaxants
- Barbiturates

NITROGEN BALANCE

Nitrogen balance refers to the difference between the daily intake and excretion of nitrogen. It is also an indicator of tissue integrity. A healthy adult experiencing a stable weight is in nitrogen equilibrium, also known as neutral nitrogen balance.

Positive nitrogen balance indicates that the intake of nitrogen exceeds excretion. Specifically, the body builds more tissue than it breaks down. This normally occurs during periods of growth: infancy, childhood, adolescence, pregnancy, and lactation.

Negative nitrogen balance indicates that the excretion of nitrogen exceeds intake. The individual is receiving insufficient protein, and the body is breaking down more tissue than it is building, as seen during periods of illness, trauma, aging, and malnutrition.

ASSESSMENT/DATA COLLECTION

- Weight and history of recent weight patterns
- Medical history for diseases that affect metabolism and nitrogen balance
- Extent of traumatic injuries, as appropriate
- Fluid and electrolyte status
- Laboratory values: albumin, transferrin, glucose, creatinine
- Clinical findings of malnutrition: pitting edema, hair loss, wasted appearance
- Medication adverse effects that can affect nutrition
- Usual 24-hr dietary intake
- Use of nutritional supplements, herbal supplements, vitamins, and minerals
- Use of alcohol, caffeine, and nicotine

NURSING INTERVENTIONS

- Monitor food intake.
- Monitor fluid intake and output.
- Use client-centered approach to address disease-specific problems with ingestion, digestion, or medication regime. ℚPCC
- Collaborate with dietitian. ℚTC
- Provide adequate calories and high-quality protein.

STRATEGIES TO INCREASE PROTEIN, CALORIC CONTENT
- Add skim milk powder to milk (double-strength milk).
- Use whole milk instead of water in recipes.
- Add cheese, peanut butter, chopped hard-boiled eggs, or yogurt to foods.
- Dip meats in eggs or milk and coat with bread crumbs before cooking.
- Nuts and dried beans are significant sources of protein. These are good alternatives for a dairy allergy or lactose intolerance.

Application Exercises

1. A nurse is discussing how the body processes food with a client during a routine provider's visit. Which of the following statements should the nurse include?

   A. Glycerol can be broken down into glucose for use by the body.

   B. The liver converts unused glucose into glycogen.

   C. Excess fatty acids are stored in the muscle tissue.

   D. The body uses glycogen for fat before using available ATP.

2. A nurse is reviewing prescribed medications for a newly admitted client. Which of the following medications increases the body's rate of metabolism?

   A. Morphine

   B. Levothyroxine

   C. Phenobarbital

   D. Dilaudid

3. A charge nurse is conducting a nutritional class for a group of newly licensed nurses regarding basal metabolic rate (BMR). The charge nurse should inform the class that which of the following factors increases BMR? (Select all that apply.)

   A. Lactation

   B. Prolonged stress

   C. Malnutrition

   D. Puberty

   E. Age older than 60 years

4. A school nurse is teaching a high school health class about the possible causes of a negative nitrogen balance. Which of the following causes should the nurse include in the teaching? (Select all that apply.)

   A. Illness

   B. Malnutrition

   C. Adolescence

   D. Trauma

   E. Pregnancy

Active Learning Scenario

A nurse is conducting a nutritional program for a group of newly licensed nurses regarding how the body uses food for energy. Use the ATI Active Learning Template: Basic Concept to complete this item.

RELATED CONTENT: Describe the steps of ingestion, digestion, and absorption.

UNDERLYING PRINCIPLES: Explain the two processes that occur during metabolism.

Application Exercises Key

1. A. Excess glycerol is reassembled with fatty acids into triglycerides.
   B. **CORRECT:** The liver converts unused glucose into glycogen, which is stored in the muscle tissue and liver for later use.
   C. Excess fatty acids are converted back to triglycerides and stored in the adipose tissue.
   D. The body uses available ATP for growth and repair, and uses stored fat and glycogen if no ATP is available.

   Ⓝ *NCLEX® Connection: Health Promotion and Maintenance, Aging Process*

2. A. Morphine is an opioid narcotic, which would decrease body metabolism.
   B. **CORRECT:** Levothyroxine is used for the treatment of hypothyroidism and increases the body's rate of metabolism.
   C. Phenobarbital is a barbiturate medication, which would decrease body metabolism.
   D. Dilaudid is an opioid narcotic, which would decrease body metabolism.

   Ⓝ *NCLEX® Connection: Physiological Adaptation, Illness Management*

3. A. **CORRECT:** Include in the teaching that lactation increases BMR.
   B. **CORRECT:** Include in the teaching that prolonged stress increases BMR.
   C. Include in the teaching that malnutrition decreases BMR.
   D. **CORRECT:** Include in the teaching that puberty increases BMR.
   E. Include in the teaching that being over 60 years of age decreases BMR.

   Ⓝ *NCLEX® Connection: Health Promotion and Maintenance, Aging Process*

4. A. **CORRECT:** Illness is a possible cause of negative nitrogen balance.
   B. **CORRECT:** Malnutrition is a possible cause of negative nitrogen balance.
   C. Adolescence is a possible cause of positive nitrogen balance.
   D. **CORRECT:** Trauma is a possible cause of negative nitrogen balance.
   E. Pregnancy is a possible cause of positive nitrogen balance.

   Ⓝ *NCLEX® Connection: Physiological Adaptation, Illness Management*

Active Learning Scenario Key

Using the ATI Active Learning Template: Basic Concept

RELATED CONTENT
- Ingestion is the process of taking in food by mouth into the digestive system.
- Digestion involves the breakdown of food into nutrients so they can be absorbed.
- Absorption is the process by which nutrients pass through the walls of the digestive system so they can be used by the body.

UNDERLYING PRINCIPLES
- Catabolism is the process by which food is broken down into small molecules to release heat and chemical energy.
- Anabolism is the formation of new body substances (tissue, bone).

Ⓝ *NCLEX® Connection: Physiologic Adaptation, Illness Management*

UNIT 1   PRINCIPLES OF NUTRITION

CHAPTER 3 # Nutrition Assessment/ Data Collection

Nurses play a key role in assessing the nutritional needs of clients. Nurses monitor and intervene with clients requiring acute and chronic nutritional care. Nurses should consider and incorporate the family's nutritional habits into a client's individual plan of care. Nurses should take an active role in assessing and teaching community groups regarding nutrition.

A collaborative, interprofessional approach provides the best outcomes for the client. Providers and nurses collect physical assessment data, as well as serving as liaison between the health care team and the dietitian. Registered dietitians complete comprehensive nutritional assessments. Nurses monitor and evaluate interventions provided to clients. Q℡

A client's physical appearance can be deceiving. A client who has a healthy weight and appearance can be malnourished. Cultural, social, and physical norms must be part of a client's assessment. Even with adequate client education, personal preferences can be an overriding factor to successful nutritional balance.

DIET HISTORY

A diet history is an assessment of usual foods, fluids, and supplements. The diet history is part of the nutrition screening performed using various settings to determine malnutrition issues. Components of the diet history include the following.

- Time, type, and amount of food eaten for breakfast, lunch, dinner, and snacks Qᴘᴄᴄ
- Time, type, and amount of fluids consumed throughout the day, including water, health drinks, coffee/tea, carbonated beverages, and beverages with caffeine
- Type, amount, and frequency of "special foods" (celebration foods, movie foods)
- Typical preparation of foods and fluids (coffee with sugar, fried foods)
- Number of meals eaten away from home (at work or school)
- Type of preferred or prescribed diet (ovo-lacto vegetarian, 2 g sodium/low-fat diet)
- Foods avoided due to allergy or preference
- Frequency and dose/amount of medications or nutritional supplements taken daily
- Satisfaction with diet over a specified time frame (last 3 months, 1 year)

TOOLS TO DETERMINE NUTRITIONAL STATUS

A physical assessment is performed by the provider or nurse to identify indicators of inadequate nutrition. However, other diseases or conditions can cause these clinical findings.

MANIFESTATIONS
- Hair that is dry or brittle, or skin that has dry patches
- Poor wound healing or sores
- Lack of subcutaneous fat or muscle wasting
- Irregular cardiovascular measurements (heart rate and rhythm, blood pressure)
- Enlarged spleen or liver
- General weakness or impaired coordination

ANTHROPOMETRIC TOOLS

Weight
- Weigh at the same time of day wearing similar clothing to ensure accurate weight readings.
- Daily fluctuations generally are indicative of water weight changes.
- Percentage weight change calculation (weight change over a specified time):

$$\% \text{ weight change} = \frac{(\text{usual weight} - \text{present weight})}{\text{usual weight}} \times 100$$

- Ideal body weight based on the Hamwi method using height/weight calculation.
  - **MALES**: 48 kg (106 lb) for the first 152 cm (5 ft) of height, and 2.7 kg (6 lb) for each additional 2.5 cm (1 in).
  - **FEMALES**: 45 kg (100 lb) for the first 152 cm (5 ft) of height, and 2.3 kg (5 lb) for each additional 2.5 cm (1 in).
- During illness, weight loss is monitored to prevent or detect malnutrition.
  - With starvation or chronic disease, weight loss indicating severe malnutrition: greater than 5%/month, greater than 7.5%/3 months, greater than 10%/6 months, greater than 20%/year
  - With acute disease or injury, weight loss indicating severe malnutrition: greater than 2%/week, greater than 5%/month, greater than 7.5%/3 months

Height
- Measure on a vertical, flat surface. Ask the client to remove shoes and head coverings and stand straight with heels together looking straight ahead. Read the measurement to the nearest 0.1 cm or 1/8 inch.
- Obtain a recumbent measurement (lying on a firm, flat surface) for infants and young children.

Body mass index (BMI)
BMI measurements compare the weight to height to estimate the effect of the individual's body weight. Client factors should be considered when determining the value of BMI measurement. For example, a client who has large muscle mass compared to height can have an increased BMI, since weight can be influenced by both fat and muscle, or a client with a normal BMI might have excess body fat.
- Healthy weight is indicated by a BMI of 18.5 to 24.9.
- Underweight is indicated by a BMI less than 18.5.
- Overweight is defined as an increased body weight in relation to height. It is indicated by a BMI of 25 to 29.9, and are about 20% above desirable levels.
- Obesity is indicated by a BMI greater than or equal to 30.

$$\text{BMI} = \text{weight (kg)} \div \text{height (m}^2\text{)}$$

CLINICAL VALUES

Fluid I&O
- Adults: 2,000 to 3,000 mL (2 to 3 L) per day
- Total average output: 1,750 to 3,000 mL/day

Protein levels are usually measured by albumin levels, although total protein is sometimes used.
- Many non-nutritional factors (injury, kidney disease), interfere with this measure for protein malnutrition.
- Expected reference range for albumin: 3.5 to 5 g/dL

Prealbumin (thyroxine-binding protein) is a sensitive measure used to assess critically ill clients who are at risk for malnutrition. This test reflects acute changes rather than gradual changes. However, it is more expensive and often unavailable. This is not part of routine assessment.
- Prealbumin levels can decrease with an inflammatory process resulting in an inaccurate measurement.
- Prealbumin levels are used to measure effectiveness of total parenteral nutrition.
- Expected reference range is 15 to 36 mg/dL. (Less than 10.7 mg/dL indicates severe nutritional deficiency.)

Nitrogen balance refers to the relationship between protein breakdown (catabolism) and protein synthesis (anabolism).
- To measure nitrogen balance
  - Record protein intake (g) over 24 hr and divide by 6.25.
  - Record nitrogen excretion in urine over 24 hr and add 4 g.
  - Subtract nitrogen output from nitrogen intake.
  - 24 hr protein intake ÷ 6.25 = nitrogen intake (g)
  - 24 hr urinary urea nitrogen + 4 g = total nitrogen output

  Nitrogen intake - total nitrogen output = nitrogen balance

- A neutral nitrogen balance indicates adequate nutritional intake.
- A positive nitrogen balance indicates protein synthesis is greater than protein breakdown as during growth, pregnancy, or during recovery.
- A negative nitrogen balance indicates protein is used at a greater rate than it is synthesized as in starvation or a catabolic state following injury or disease.

Obesity

Approximately 36.5% of American adults have obesity, and an estimated 68.5% have obesity or are overweight.
- Obesity is a chronic condition caused by calorie intake in excess of energy expenditure. It can be affected by numerous factors (culture, metabolism, environment, socioeconomics, individual behaviors).
- Obesity might be linked to protective measures within the body to prevent weight loss during calorie restriction, which cause it to secrete hormones that stimulate the appetite to maintain a specific weight. As weight increases, the body accepts a higher weight as the expected weight and seeks to maintain it.

ASSESSMENT

RISK FACTORS

- Genetic predisposition
- Hormones (leptin, ghrelin)
- Behavioral factors (sedentary lifestyle, diet choices)

EXPECTED FINDINGS

Clients report of depression, low self-esteem, avoidance of health-related appointments, and no desire to exercise as a result of feeling stigmatized by their excessive weight

Body mass index
- Overweight: 25 to 29.9
- Obesity: 30 or greater

Waist circumference
- Females: greater than 88.9 cm (35 in)
- Males: greater than 101.6 cm (40 in)

Waist-to-hip ratio (WHR)
- Measurement of difference between peripheral lower body obesity and central obesity
- Can be used as a predictor of coronary artery disease
- Indicates excess fat at the waist and abdomen
  - Males: 0.95 or greater
  - Females: 0.8 or greater

LABORATORY TESTS

- Screening to evaluate for cardiovascular disease, diabetes mellitus, fatty liver disease, or thyroid disorders
- Total cholesterol
- Triglycerides
- Fasting blood glucose
- Glycosylated hemoglobin
- Aspartate aminotransferase (AST)
- Alanine aminotransferase (ALT)

PATIENT-CENTERED CARE

MEDICATIONS

- Clients who do not lose weight during weight loss programs can benefit from pharmacological therapy.
- Anorectic medications suppress appetite and reduce food intake. When combined with an exercise program, they can result in weight loss.

Orlistat

Prevents digestion of fats

ADVERSE EFFECTS: Oily discharge; reduced food and vitamin absorption; decreased bile flow; loose, oily stools; abdominal cramps; fecal incontinence

Lorcaserin

Stimulates serotonin receptors in the hypothalamus in the brain to curb appetite

ADVERSE EFFECTS: Headache, dry mouth, fatigue, nausea

Phentermine-topiramate

Suppresses the appetite and induces a feeling of satiety.

ADVERSE EFFECTS: Dry mouth, constipation, nausea, change in taste, dizziness, insomnia, numbness and tingling of extremities

CONTRAINDICATIONS: Hyperthyroidism, glaucoma, taking an MAO inhibitor

INTERPROFESSIONAL CARE

The care team can include a health care provider, nursing team, dietitian, social worker, surgeon, and mental health therapist or counselor.

NURSING CARE

- Maintain low-Fowler's position to maximize chest expansion.
- Monitor respiratory status frequently and include pulse oximetry continuously.
- Supplement oxygen as needed.
- Monitor blood pressure, using an appropriately-sized cuff for accurate readings.
- Monitor frequently for medication adverse effects.
- Use bariatric equipment (lifts, transport equipment, beds) to assist in mobility as needed.

CLIENT EDUCATION: Follow the prescribed diet from the provider or dietitian to prevent complications of obesity.

SURGICAL INTERVENTIONS

Bariatric surgery

SEE AMS CHAPTER 47: GASTROINTESTINAL THERAPEUTIC PROCEDURES.

COMPLICATIONS

- Obesity increases the risk for dyslipidemia, diabetes mellitus type 2, vascular disease, gallbladder disease, hypertension, osteoarthritis, respiratory problems, some cancers, and sleep apnea.
- Obesity also increases the risk for perioperative complications and complications during pregnancy, labor, and delivery.

Reduced life expectancy

- For class I obesity, life expectancy is reduced by 2 to 4 years.
- For BMI 40 to 50, life expectancy is reduced by 8 to 10 years.

Other complications

Nonalcoholic fatty liver disease, polycystic ovary syndrome, gastroesophageal reflux disease

RISK FACTORS FOR INADEQUATE NUTRITION

BIOPHYSICAL FACTORS
- Medical disease/conditions (hypertension, HIV/AIDS)
- Preventive measures or disease treatments, including surgery or use of medications and supplements.
- Genetic predisposition (lactose intolerance, osteoporosis)
- Age

PSYCHOLOGICAL FACTORS
- Mental illness (clinical depression)
- Excessive stress
- Negative self-concept
- Use of comfort foods

SOCIOECONOMIC FACTORS
- Poverty
- Alcohol and other substance use disorders
- Fad or "special" diets
- Food preferences: cultural, ethnic, or religious

Active Learning Scenario

A community health nurse is conducting a dietary assessment for a client. Use the ATI Active Learning Template: Basic Concept to complete this item.

UNDERLYING PRINCIPLES: Describe four components of a diet history.

EFFECT OF RISK FACTORS ON NUTRITIONAL STATUS

The following are examples of how risk factors can affect nutritional status.
- A client who has edema can require treatment with a diuretic and low-sodium diet. Diuretics can cause sodium and potassium imbalances. A low-sodium diet can be unappetizing and cause the client to eat less.
- Osteoporosis has many modifiable risk factors. A client who takes action to prevent osteoporosis (increasing intake of vitamin D and calcium, engaging in weight-bearing exercise, reducing use of tobacco and alcohol products) will positively affect their nutritional status.
- Poor self-concept can cause a client to avoid eating or to overeat.

NURSING ACTIONS
- In addition to determining the client's nutrient and calorie intake, assess other factors that might alter nutrient intake.
- Consult with the provider to see if the client's medical treatment plan needs to be altered to improve nutrition, such as administering a different medication to prevent the adverse effect of anorexia, or adding a medication to treat nausea or improve appetite.
- Plan the client's schedule of activities to prevent interruptions during mealtime, and to avoid fatigue, nausea, or pain before meals.

Application Exercises

1. A nurse in a nutrition clinic is calculating body mass index (BMI) for several clients. The nurse should identify which of the following client BMIs as overweight?

   A. 24

   B. 30

   C. 27

   D. 32

2. A nurse on an orthopedic unit is reviewing data for a client who sustained trauma in a motor-vehicle crash. Which of the following values indicates the client is in a catabolic state (using protein faster than protein is being synthesized)?

   A. Blood albumin 3.5 g/dL

   B. Negative nitrogen balance

   C. BMI of 18.5

   D. Blood prealbumin 15 mg/dL

3. A nurse is performing a nutrition assessment on a client. Which of the following clinical findings are suggestive of malnutrition? (Select all that apply.)

   A. Poor wound healing

   B. Dry hair

   C. Blood pressure 130/80 mm Hg

   D. Weak hand grips

   E. Impaired coordination

4. A nurse is teaching a group of female clients about risk factors for developing osteoporosis. Which of the following risk factors should the nurse include? (Select all that apply.)

   A. Inactivity

   B. Family history

   C. Obesity

   D. Hyperlipidemia

   E. Cigarette smoking

Application Exercises Key

1. A. A healthy weight is indicated by a BMI of 18.5 to 24.9.
   B. Obesity is an excess amount of body fat indicated by a BMI greater than or equal to 30.
   C. **CORRECT:** Overweight is defined as an increased body weight in relation to height, indicated by a BMI of 25 to 29.9.
   D. Obesity is an excess amount of body fat indicated by a BMI greater than or equal to 30.

   Ⓝ *NCLEX® Connection: Basic Care and Comfort, Nutrition and Oral Hydration*

2. A. Blood albumin levels reflect slow changes in protein levels, not acute. An albumin level of 3.5 g/dL or 4.5 g/dL is within the expected reference range.
   B. **CORRECT:** A negative nitrogen balance indicates protein is used at a greater rate than it is synthesized as in starvation or a catabolic state following injury or disease.
   C. A BMI of 18.5 indicates an ideal body weight.
   D. A blood prealbumin of 15 mg/dL is within the expected reference range.

   Ⓝ *NCLEX® Connection: Reduction of Risk Potential, Laboratory Values*

3. A. **CORRECT:** Poor wound healing describes changes reflective of malnutrition.
   B. **CORRECT:** Dry hair describes changes reflective of malnutrition.
   C. A blood pressure value of 130/80 mm Hg is an expected cardiovascular finding and is not associated with malnutrition.
   D. **CORRECT:** Weak hand grips describe changes reflective of malnutrition.
   E. **CORRECT:** Impaired coordination describes changes reflective of malnutrition.

   Ⓝ *NCLEX® Connection: Basic Care and Comfort, Nutrition and Oral Hydration*

4. A. **CORRECT:** There is an increased risk for osteoporosis due to inactivity. Weight-bearing exercises are a primary prevention measure.
   B. **CORRECT:** A family history of osteoporosis is a risk factor.
   C. Weight loss can cause a decreased intake of dietary calcium and vitamin D, leading to the development of osteoporosis.
   D. Hyperlipidemia is not a risk factor for the development of osteoporosis in females.
   E. **CORRECT:** Cigarette smoking can increase the incidence of osteoporosis.

   Ⓝ *NCLEX® Connection: Health Promotion and Maintenance, Health Promotion/Disease Prevention*

Active Learning Scenario Key

Using the ATI Active Learning Template: Basic Concept

UNDERLYING PRINCIPLES: A diet history is an assessment of usual foods, fluids, and supplements.

- Time, type, and amount of food eaten for breakfast, lunch, dinner, and snacks.
- Time, type, and amount of fluids consumed throughout the day including water, health drinks, coffee/tea, carbonated beverages, and beverages with caffeine.
- Type, amount, and frequency of "special foods" (celebration foods, movie foods).
- Typical preparation of foods and fluids (coffee with sugar, fried foods).
- Number of meals eaten away from home (at work or school).
- Type of diet (ovo-lacto vegetarian, 2 g sodium/low-fat diet).
- Foods avoided due to allergy or preference.
- Frequency and dose/amount of medications or nutritional supplements taken daily.
- Satisfaction with diet over a specified time frame (last 3 months, year).

Ⓝ *NCLEX® Connection: Health Promotion and Maintenance, Health Screening*

CHAPTER 4

Guidelines for Healthy Eating

Nutrition is vital to maintaining optimal health. Healthy food choices and controlling weight are important steps in promoting health and reducing risk factors for disease.

Nurses should encourage favorable nutritional choices and can serve as informational resources for clients regarding guidelines for healthy eating.

Established guidelines for healthy eating that clients and nurses can refer to include the Dietary Guidelines for Americans and MyPlate, along with a number of condition- or system-specific guidelines.

Vegetarian diets can meet all nutrient recommendations. It is essential to consume a variety and correct amount of foods to meet individual caloric needs.

DIETARY GUIDELINES FOR AMERICANS

- The U.S. Department of Agriculture (USDA) and the U.S. Department of Health and Human Services (HHS) publish the Dietary Guidelines for Americans jointly every 5 years. These guidelines are based on evidence-based advice concerning food intake and physical activity for Americans older than 2 years of age, including those at risk for chronic disease. The updates can be found on the USDA and health.gov websites.
- The Dietary Guidelines for Americans advocates healthy food selections: a variety of fiber-rich fruits and vegetables, whole grains, low-fat or fat-free milk and milk products, lean meats, poultry, fish, legumes, eggs, and nuts. Recommendations include nutrient-dense foods and beverages.
  - Balance energy intake with energy expenditure by selecting a wide variety of foods, and limiting saturated and trans saturated fat, sugars, sodium, and alcohol.
  - Establish exercise routines to promote cardiovascular health, muscle strength and endurance, and psychological well-being.
  - Consume a minimum of five servings per day of fiber-rich fruits and vegetables to in order to decrease risk factors for some cancers. The vitamin and mineral content of these foods can also decrease the risk of DNA damage.
  - Choose monounsaturated and polyunsaturated fats from fish, lean meats, nuts, and vegetable oils. Fat intake can average 30% of total caloric intake with a goal of less than 7% from saturated fats. While progressing toward the 7% goal, individuals should try to consume less than 10% of intake from saturated fats, and progress to 7% or less over time.
  - Limit sugar and starchy foods to decrease the risk of dental caries.
  - Consume less than 2,300 mg/day (about 1 tsp) of salt by limiting most canned and processed foods. Prepare foods without adding salt. Middle-aged and older adults benefit even more from a diet with 1,500 mg/day or less of sodium.
  - Drink alcohol in moderation: up to one drink per day for females and two per day for males. Some medical conditions, medication therapies, and physical activities preclude the use of alcohol.
  - Eating at least 12 oz seafood from a variety of sources is beneficial for individuals older than age 12 years who are not pregnant or nursing. Observe local seafood advisories closely, and limit consumption of large, predatory fish.
  - Follow food safety guidelines when preparing, cooking, and storing food. Avoid consumption of raw eggs and unpasteurized milk and juices. Qs
- These strategies are beneficial for cooking foods at home.
  - When using convenience foods or boxed meals, add healthy ingredients (frozen vegetables, canned legumes) to increase the volume of food and add nutrition.
  - Decrease the amount of salt or seasonings containing sodium when cooking.
  - Buy side items that increase the nutritional value of meals (packaged salad kits, pre-cut fruit, whole-grain bread).
- When eating out, these strategies can help meet nutritional guidelines.
  - Eat a high-fiber snack 1 hour before leaving to eat. It is easier to make healthier food choices when not really hungry.
  - If one meal out is going to be high-calorie, make the other meals of the day lower in calories and high in nutrients and fiber to provide balance.
  - Watch for components that add fat content to the meal (fatty meats, nuts, creams, gravies and sauces with whole milk, fatty salad dressings). Asking for these items on the side can reduce the amount consumed.
  - Pick restaurants that offer healthy options.

MYPLATE

The USDA sponsors a website that promotes healthy food choices balanced with physical activity (www.choosemyplate.gov). MyPlate is based on the current USDA dietary guidelines, and is a tool to help individuals identify daily amounts of foods based on criteria (age, sex, activity level). The food groups represented are grains, vegetables, fruit, dairy, oils, and protein foods.

MyPlate can serve as a reminder to balance calorie intake with suitable activity.

- Adults should engage in at least 2.5 hr/week of moderate-level aerobic physical activity or 1.25 hr/week of vigorous aerobic physical activity.
- Children and adolescents should be physically active for 60 min/day, the majority of which should be moderate or vigorous aerobic physical activity, but developmentally appropriate and fun. Children should engage in muscle strengthening activities at least 3 days/week. Activity levels can be met in short periods of activity throughout the day instead of a sustained 60 min.
- The MyPlate image and information sheet are available in multiple languages to assist with client education.

VEGETARIAN DIETS

- A vegetarian diet focuses on plants for food, including fruits, vegetables, dried beans and peas, grains, seeds, and nuts. There is no single type of vegetarian diet. Vegetarian eating patterns usually fall into the following groups.
  - **Vegan** diet excludes all meat and animal products.
  - **Lacto vegetarian** diet includes dairy products.
  - **Lacto-ovo vegetarian** diet includes dairy products and eggs.
- People who follow vegetarian diets can get all the nutrients they need, but they must be careful to eat a wide variety of foods to meet their nutritional needs. It is important to discuss ensuring enough vitamin D and B$_{12}$, calcium, and omega-3 fatty acids are consumed by clients who follow a vegan diet.

FOOD LABELS

- The Food and Drug Administration (FDA) requires certain information be included with packaged foods and beverages. The information is included on the nutrition facts label or food label, which is a boxed label found on foods and beverages. Food labels must include single serving size, number of servings in the package, percent of daily values, and the amount of each nutrient in one serving.
- The Percent Daily Values information is typically based on a 2,000 calorie/day diet, but for certain nutrients and food components can be based on 2,500 calorie/day.

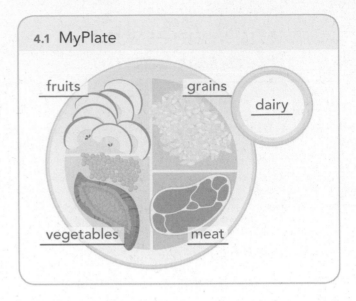

4.1 MyPlate

NUTRIENTS INCLUDED ON THE FOOD LABEL

- Calories
- Calories from fat
- Total fat
- Saturated fat
- Trans fat
- Cholesterol
- Sodium
- Total carbohydrates
- Dietary fiber
- Sugars
- Protein
- Vitamin D
- Potassium
- Calcium
- Iron
- Foods marketed as functional foods might be whole foods or foods with additives (herbs, minerals). These foods are often advertised as having the ability to prevent or promote disease. There is no regulation regarding functional foods at this time.
- Organic food products are regulated under the USDA.
  - Organic foods are produced without the use of pesticide or synthetic fertilizer.
  - Organic livestock must be fed organic feed during pregnancy for a specific time period and cannot receive growth hormones, antibiotics, or other medications.
- Organic foods might help prevent pathogen resistance to antibiotics. While they reduce exposure to pesticides, there is no evidence that it has a healthy effect. Clarify misinformation about these foods with clients.

CLIENT EDUCATION

- Read food labels properly (comparing nutrient, calorie, fat, and sodium levels) to ensure individual nutritional needs are met, and healthy choices are made.
- Goods that are genetically engineered or contain genetically modified organisms (GMO) have not been proven harmful.

4.2 MyPlate recommended servings

RECOMMENDED DAILY SERVINGS			FOOD SOURCES
Grains			

Whole grains should equal half of the grains eaten.

Children	Females	Males	
2 to 3 years: 3 oz	9 to 13 years: 5 oz	9 to 13 years: 3 oz	One slice bread = 1 oz
4 to 8 years: 5 oz	14 to 50 years: 6 oz	14 to 18 years: 4 oz	1 cup flake cereal = 1 oz
	51 years and older: 5 oz	19 to 30 years: 8 oz	½ cup cooked pasta = 1 oz
		31 to 50 years: 7 oz	1 6-inch flour tortilla = 1 oz
		51 years and older: 6 oz	

Vegetables			

Vegetables include raw, cooked, frozen, canned, dried, or 100% juice.

Children	Females	Males	Broccoli, carrots, pumpkin, tomato juice, peas, corn, potatoes, onions, mushrooms
2 to 3 years: 1 cup	9 to 13 years: 2 cups	9 to 13 years: 2.5 cups	
4 to 8 years: 1.5 cups	14 to 50 years: 2.5 cups	14 to 50 years: 3 cups	
	51 years and older: 2 cups	51 years and older: 2.5 cups	

Fruits			

Fruits include fresh, frozen, canned, dried, or 100% juice.

Children	Females	Males	
2 to 3 years: 1 cup	9 to 18 years: 1.5 cups	9 to 13 years: 1.5 cups	One small banana – ½ cup serving
4 to 8 years: 1 to 1.5 cups	19 to 30 years: 2 cups	14 years and older: 2 cups	One small orange = ½ cup serving
	31 years and older: 1.5 cups		¼ cup dried apricots = ½ cup serving

Dairy			

Dairy selections should include reduced-fat or fat-free options. Higher-fat options are counted as part of daily calories from solid fats and added sugars (i.e., empty calories).

Children	Females and Males		Milk, yogurt, cheese, pudding, ice cream, soy milk
2 to 3 years: 2 cups	9 years and older: 3 cups		¼ cup evaporated milk = 1 cup serving
4 to 8 years: 2.5 cups			½ cup shredded cheese = 1 cup serving
			1.5 oz hard cheese = 1 cup serving
			½ cup ricotta cheese = 1 cup serving
			2 cups cottage cheese = 1 cup serving
			1.5 cups ice cream = 1 cup serving

Proteins			

Protein requirements can increase with physical activity. Selection should include lean or low-fat proteins. Higher fat options are counted as part of daily calories from solid fats and added sugars (i.e., empty calories).

Children	Females	Males	Meats (beef, pork), poultry, eggs, kidney beans, soy beans, seafood, nuts and seeds, peanut butter
2 to 3 years: 2 oz	9 to 18 years: 5 oz	9 to 13 years: 5 oz	One small chicken breast = 3 oz
4 to 8 years: 4 oz	19 to 30 years: 5.5 oz	14 to 30 years: 6.5 oz	1 can drained tuna = 3 to 4 oz
	31 years and older: 5 oz	31 to 50 years: 6 oz	One egg = 1 oz
		51 years and older: 5.5 oz	¼ cup cooked beans = 1 oz
			½ oz seeds or nuts = 1 oz

Oils			

Children	Females	Males	Vegetable oils (canola, corn, olive, peanut, safflower, soybean, sunflower), mayonnaise, some salad dressings, avocado, nuts and seeds
2 to 3 years: 3 tsp	9 to 18 years: 5 tsp	9 to 13 years: 5 tsp	
4 to 8 years: 4 tsp	19 to 30 years: 6 tsp	14 to 18 year: 6 tsp	
	31 years and older: 5 tsp	19 to 30 years: 7 tsp	Avocados and olives are also part of the vegetable food group.
		31 years and older: 6 tsp	Nuts and seeds are also part of the protein food group.

STRATEGIES FOR PROMOTION OF SPECIFIC AREAS OF HEALTH

Heart

- Limit saturated fat to 10% of calories. Consume as little cholesterol in the diet as possible, as long as it does not hinder a healthy eating pattern.
- For individuals with elevated low density lipoprotein (LDL), the American Heart Association (AHA) recommends increasing monounsaturated fats and soluble fiber.
- The Dietary Approaches to Stop Hypertension (DASH) diet is proven by research to significantly lower systolic and diastolic blood pressure. Q EBP

Nervous system

- Normal functioning of the nervous system depends on adequate levels of the B-complex vitamins, especially thiamin, niacin, and vitamins B_6 and B_{12}.
- Calcium and sodium are important regulators of nerve responses. Consuming the recommended servings from the grain and dairy food groups provides these nutrients.

Bones

- Consuming the recommended servings from the MyPlate's dairy group supplies the calcium, magnesium, and phosphorus necessary for bone formation.
- Weight-bearing physical activity is essential to decrease the risk of osteoporosis.

Bowel function

- Normal bowel functioning depends on adequate fluid intake and 25 g/day of fiber for females, and 38 g/day for males.
- The minimum number of servings from MyPlate's fruit, vegetable, and grain food groups (specifically whole grains) provides the essential nutrients.

Cancer prevention

- A well-balanced diet using MyPlate and a healthy weight are guidelines to prevent cancer.
- Increase high-fiber plant-based foods.
- Limit saturated and trans fat, while emphasizing foods with polyunsaturated fats (omega-3 fatty acids).
- Limit sodium intake.
- Avoid excess alcohol intake.
- Include regular physical activity.

Active Learning Scenario

A community health nurse is conducting a nutritional class regarding cancer prevention strategies. Use the ATI Active Learning Template: Basic Concept to complete this item.

RELATED CONTENT: Describe four components recommended to prevent cancer.

Application Exercises

1. A nurse is providing teaching to a client who follows vegan dietary practices. The nurse should instruct the client that there is a risk of having a deficit in which of the following nutrients? (Select all that apply.)
   A. Vitamin D
   B. Fiber
   C. Calcium
   D. Vitamin B_{12}
   E. Whole grains

2. A nurse is conducting a nutrition class at a local community center. Which of the following information should the nurse include in the teaching?
   A. Progress toward limiting saturated fat to 7% of total daily intake.
   B. Good bowel function requires 35 g/day of fiber for females.
   C. Limit cholesterol consumption to 400 mg/day.
   D. Normal functioning cardiac systems depends on B-complex vitamins.

3. A nurse is discussing essential nutrients for normal functioning of the nervous system with a client. Which of the following should the nurse include in the teaching? (Select all that apply.)
   A. Calcium
   B. Thiamin
   C. Vitamin B_6
   D. Sodium
   E. Phosphorus

4. A school nurse is teaching a group of students how to read food labels. Which of the following is a required component of food labels that the nurse should include in the teaching? (Select all that apply.)
   A. Total carbohydrates
   B. Total fat
   C. Calories
   D. Magnesium
   E. Dietary fiber

Application Exercises Key

1. A. **CORRECT:** Instruct the client to ensure an adequate consumption of vitamin D because most dietary vitamin D is consumed via fortified milk products. The vegan diet includes plant foods, and excludes all animal-derived products.
   B. Because the vegan diet consists of plant foods, adequate fiber consumption is not a concern. Fiber is found primarily in plants.
   C. **CORRECT:** Instruct the client to monitor and ensure an adequate consumption of calcium because there are few good sources of calcium from plant sources. The vegan diet excludes all animal-derived products.
   D. **CORRECT:** Instruct the client to ensure they are consuming adequate vitamin B_{12} because all reliable sources of vitamin B_{12} are in animal products. The vegan diet excludes all animal-derived products.
   E. Because the vegan diet consists of plant foods, adequate consumption of whole grains is not a concern. Grains are included as part of the vegan diet.

   Ⓝ *NCLEX® Connection: Health Promotion and Maintenance, Health Promotion/Disease Prevention*

2. A. **CORRECT:** Include for the clients to progress toward limiting saturated fat to 7% of total daily intake.
   B. Good bowel function requires 25 g/day of fiber for females, and 38 g/day for males.
   C. Cholesterol consumption should be limited to between 200 and 300 mg/day.
   D. Normal functioning nervous system, instead of cardiac, depends on B-complex vitamins.

   Ⓝ *NCLEX® Connection: Health Promotion and Maintenance, Health Promotion/Disease Prevention*

3. A. **CORRECT:** Calcium is an important regulator of nerve responses.
   B. **CORRECT:** Normal functioning of the nervous system depends on adequate levels of the B-complex vitamins, especially thiamin, niacin, and vitamins B_6 and B_{12}.
   C. **CORRECT:** Normal functioning of the nervous system depends on adequate levels of the B-complex vitamins, especially thiamin, niacin, and vitamins B_6 and B_{12}.
   D. **CORRECT:** Sodium is an important regulator of nerve responses.
   E. Phosphorus helps maintain acid-base balance, as well as formation of bone and teeth, and does not directly affect functioning of the nervous system.

   Ⓝ *NCLEX® Connection: Health Promotion and Maintenance, Health Promotion/Disease Prevention*

4. A. **CORRECT:** The Food and Drug Administration (FDA) requires certain information be included with packaged foods and beverages. Total carbohydrates are included on food labels.
   B. **CORRECT:** Food labels must include single serving size, number of servings in the package, percent of daily values, and the amount of each nutrient in one serving. Total fat is included on food labels.
   C. **CORRECT:** Calories are included on food labels.
   D. Magnesium is not included on food labels.
   E. **CORRECT:** Dietary fiber is included on food labels.

   Ⓝ *NCLEX® Connection: Health Promotion and Maintenance, Aging Process*

Active Learning Scenario Key

Using the ATI Active Learning Template: Basic Concept
RELATED CONTENT

A well-balanced diet using the MyPlate and a healthy weight are guidelines to prevent cancer.
- Increase high-fiber plant-based foods.
- Limit saturated and polyunsaturated fat while emphasizing foods with monounsaturated fat or omega-3 fatty acids (nuts and fish).
- Limit sodium intake.
- Avoid excess alcohol intake.
- Include regular physical activity.

Ⓝ *NCLEX® Connection: Health Promotion and Maintenance, Health Promotion/Disease Prevention*

CHAPTER 5

Food Safety

Food safety is an important concept in nursing. It is essential to provide clients with the necessary education regarding food safety and food-medication interactions.

Food safety concerns include preventing aspiration of food, reducing the risk of foodborne illness, assessing for food allergies, and understanding food-medication interactions.

FOOD SAFETY GUIDELINES

Ingestion of food poses a risk of aspiration in some circumstances.
- To minimize the risk of aspiration, food should be consumed only by individuals who are conscious and have an intact gag or swallow reflex. Qs
- For clients who have a known risk of aspiration (following a stroke or a procedure involving anesthesia of the esophagus), it is important for nurses to monitor the client's ability to swallow prior to eating.
- Young children are at an increased risk for aspiration of some foods.

FOOD SAFETY REQUIREMENTS
- Proper food storage
- Proper handling
- Proper preparation

FOOD STORAGE GUIDELINES

Fresh meat: Maintain refrigerator temperature at 40° F (4° C) or colder.
- **Bacon:** 7 days
- **Sausage** (pork/chicken/beef/turkey): 1 to 2 days
- **Summer sausage:** 3 months (unopened); 3 weeks (opened)
- **Steaks, chops, roasts** (beef, veal, lamb, or pork): 3 to 5 days
- **Chicken or turkey** (whole/parts): 1 to 2 days
- **Fish:** Maintain refrigerator temperature at 40° F (4° C) or colder.
  - Lean or fatty: 1 to 2 days
  - Smoked: 14 days
  - Fresh shellfish: 1 to 2 days
  - Canned: 3 to 4 days (after opening); 5 years (pantry)

Eggs: Store in the refrigerator for 4 to 5 weeks in shell, and 1 week if hard-boiled.

Fruits and vegetables: Refrigerate perishable fruits and vegetables at 40° F (4° C). All pre-cut and pre-peeled fruits and vegetables should also be refrigerated.

Perishables: Do not leave at room temperature for more than 2 hr (1 hr if the temperature is 90° F [32° C] or above).

Canned goods: Check for rusting, crushing, and denting. Observe for stickiness on the outside of can, which can indicate leakage. Do not use any canned foods that are damaged.

HANDLING GUIDELINES

- Wash hands and food preparation surfaces frequently, and before handling food.
- Separate foods to avoid cross-contamination.

PREPARATION GUIDELINES

Cook food to the proper temperature followed by a 3-min rest time.
- Roasts and steaks: 145° F (63° C)
- Chicken: 165° F (74° C)
- Ground beef: 160° F (71° C)
- Products that contain eggs: 160° F (71° C)

PACKAGING LABELS
- **Sell-by date:** The final recommended day of sale.
- **Use-by date:** How long the product will maintain top quality.
- **Expiration date:** The final day the product should be used or consumed.

FOODBORNE ILLNESS

Foodborne illnesses occur due to improper storage of food products, as well as unsafe handling and preparation. In order to decrease the incidence of foodborne illnesses, primary education should be conducted by nurses. Proper handing and preparation is simple and includes performing frequent hand hygiene. It is important to refrigerate food products when necessary, and to avoid cross-contamination when preparing food. Food should be heated to recommended temperatures to kill unwanted bacteria. Following these basic principles can prevent the occurrence of foodborne illnesses. Qs
- Foodborne illnesses pose the greatest risk to children, older adults, immunocompromised clients, and pregnant clients. Ⓖ
- Viruses cause the majority of foodborne illnesses, but bacteria are responsible for the majority of deaths caused by foodborne illness.
- Foods most commonly associated with foodborne illness are the following.
  - Raw or undercooked foods of animal origin
  - Raw fruits and vegetables contaminated with animal feces
  - Raw sprouts
  - Unpasteurized fruit juice and milk products
  - Uncooked food handled by someone who is ill

COMMON FOODBORNE ILLNESSES

Bacterial

Salmonella: Occurs due to eating undercooked or raw meat, poultry, eggs, fish, fruit, and dairy products. Common manifestations include headache, fever, abdominal cramping, diarrhea, nausea, and vomiting. This condition can be fatal.

Escherichia coli 0157:H7: Raw or undercooked meat, especially ground beef, can cause this foodborne pathogen. Findings include severe abdominal pain and diarrhea. The pathogen can also cause hemolytic uremic syndrome, which manifests as severe anemia and kidney failure.

Listeria monocytogenes: Soft cheese, raw milk products, undercooked poultry, processed meats, and raw vegetables can cause the illness. *Listeria monocytogenes* causes significant problems for newborns, pregnant clients, and immunocompromised clients. Onset occurs with the development of a sudden fever, diarrhea, headache, back pain, and abdominal discomfort. It can lead to stillbirth or miscarriage.

Viral

Norovirus: A viral infection caused by consuming contaminated fruits and vegetables, salads prepared by someone who is infected, oysters, and contaminated water. Norovirus is very contagious, and has an onset of 24 to 48 hr. Manifestations include projectile vomiting, fever, myalgia, watery diarrhea, and headache.

FOOD ALLERGIES

Nutritional assessment/data collection includes identification of food allergies. A food allergy is a reaction that will occur each time the client is exposed to the food and initiate release of serotonin and histamine. Food intolerances do not occur consistently and are dependent on the amount of food eaten.

- Milk, peanuts, fish, eggs, soy, shellfish, tree nuts, and wheat are the most commonly reported food allergies in adults. Some infants exhibit an allergic reaction to cow's milk and/or soy, but typically outgrow this by 4 years of age.
- Common manifestations of food allergy include nausea, vomiting, diarrhea, abdominal distention, and pain. Some reactions are severe and can cause anaphylaxis.

FOOD-MEDICATION INTERACTIONS

Foods and medications can interact in the body in ways that alter the intended action of medications. The composition and timing of food intake should be considered in relation to medication use.

Foods can alter the absorption of medications.
- **Increased absorption:** Improves the peak effects of some drugs when taken with food.
- **Decreased absorption:** Food can decrease the rate and extent of absorption.
  - Reducing the rate of absorption delays the onset of peak effects.
  - Reducing the extent of absorption reduces the intended effect of the medication.

Some medications cause gastric irritation. It is important to take those medications (ibuprofen, amoxicillin, some antidepressants [bupropion]) with food to avoid gastric upset.

Some foods alter the metabolism/actions of medications. Qs
- Grapefruit juice interferes with the metabolism of many medications, resulting in an increased blood level of the medication.
- Foods high in vitamin K (dark green vegetables, eggs, carrots) can decrease the anticoagulant effects of warfarin.
- Foods high in protein can increase the metabolism of the anti-Parkinson's medication levodopa, which decreases the medication's absorption and amount transported to the brain.
- Tyramine is a naturally occurring amine found in many foods that has hypertensive effects similar to other amines (norepinephrine). Tyramine is metabolized by MAO, and clients taking MAOIs (phenelzine, selegiline) who consume foods high in tyramine can suffer a hypertensive crisis. Foods high in tyramine include aged cheese, smoked meats, dried fish, and overripe avocados.
- Herbal supplements can cause potential interactions with prescribed medications. It is important that any herbal medication consumed by a client be discussed with the provider.

NURSING ASSESSMENT/DATA COLLECTION AND INTERVENTIONS

- Nursing assessments should include a complete dietary profile of the client, medications, herbal supplements, baseline knowledge about food safety, and food-medication interactions.
- Nursing interventions should include basic teaching about food safety, and the interactions between food and client medications.
- Teach the client about the difference between food intolerance and food allergy.

Application Exercises

1. A nurse is teaching about food safety and foodborne illness to a group of adults at a local community center. Which of the following information should the nurse include?

   A. "Unpasteurized fruit juice is a common cause of foodborne illness."

   B. "Store hard-boiled eggs in the refrigerator for up to 2 weeks."

   C. "The recommended cooking temperature for ground beef is 145° F."

   D. "The onset of norovirus is 5 to 7 days after exposure to the bacteria."

2. A nurse is providing teaching about food allergies to a group of new parents. Infants who react to which of the following foods typically outgrow the sensitivity? (Select all that apply.)

   A. Soy

   B. Wheat

   C. Cow's milk

   D. Eggs

   E. Fish

3. A nurse is providing teaching to a client who is to begin taking phenelzine. Consuming which of the following foods while taking this medication could cause a hypertensive crisis?

   A. Grapefruit juice

   B. Dark green vegetables

   C. Greek yogurt

   D. Smoked fish

Active Learning Scenario

A nurse is providing teaching to a client about food safety. What should the nurse include in the teaching? Use the ATI Active Learning Template: Basic Concept to complete this item.

UNDERLYING PRINCIPLES

- Describe four food storage guidelines.
- Describe three foodborne illnesses and how they are acquired.

Application Exercises Key

1. A. **CORRECT:** Include in the teaching that unpasteurized fruit juice is a common cause of foodborne illness. Other common causes of foodborne illness include raw or undercooked foods of animal origin, raw fruits and vegetables contaminated with animal feces, and uncooked food handled by someone who is ill.
    B. Include in the teaching to store hard-boiled eggs no longer than 1 week.
    C. Include in the teaching that the recommended cooking temperature for ground beef is 160° F (71° C).
    D. Include in the teaching that the onset of norovirus is 24 to 48 hr after exposure to the virus.

    Ⓝ *NCLEX® Connection: Health Promotion and Maintenance, Aging Process*

2. A. **CORRECT:** Infants who react to soy typically outgrow the sensitivity by the age of 4 years.
    B. Include in the teaching that wheat is a common food allergy, but do not include that sensitivities during infancy are typically outgrown later in life.
    C. **CORRECT:** Infants who react to cow's milk typically outgrow the sensitivity by the age of 4 years.
    D. Include in the teaching that eggs are a common food allergy, but do not include that sensitivities during infancy are typically outgrown later in life.
    E. Include in the teaching that fish is a common food allergy, but do not include that sensitivities during infancy are typically outgrown later in life.

    Ⓝ *NCLEX® Connection: Health Promotion and Maintenance, Aging Process*

3. A. Grapefruit juice interferes with the metabolism of many medications, but will not cause a hypertensive crisis in the client who is taking phenelzine.
    B. Dark green vegetables can decrease the anticoagulant effects of warfarin, but will not cause a hypertensive crisis in the client who is taking phenelzine.
    C. Greek yogurt is a source of protein that can increase the metabolism of levodopa, but will not cause a hypertensive crisis in the client who is taking phenelzine.
    D. **CORRECT:** Smoked fish is high in tyramine, which has hypertensive effects similar to other amines. Because tyramine is metabolized by MAO, clients who are taking MAOIs (phenelzine) and consume tyramine can experience a hypertensive crisis.

    Ⓝ *NCLEX® Connection: Basic Care and Comfort, Nutrition and Oral Hydration*

Active Learning Scenario Key

Using the ATI Active Learning Template: Basic Concept

UNDERLYING PRINCIPLES

- Proper food storage guidelines
  - Fresh meat: Maintain refrigerator temperature at 40° F (4° C) or colder.
    - Bacon: 7 days
    - Sausage (pork/chicken/beef/turkey): 1 to 2 days
    - Summer sausage: 3 months (unopened); 3 weeks (opened)
    - Steaks, chops, roasts (beef, veal, lamb, or pork): 3 to 5 days
    - Chicken or turkey (whole/parts): 1 to 2 days
  - Fish: Maintain refrigerator temperature at 40° F (4° C) or colder.
    - Lean or fatty: 1 to 2 days
    - Smoked: 14 days
    - Fresh shellfish: 1 to 2 days
    - Canned: 3 to 4 days (after opening); 5 years (pantry)
  - Eggs: Store in the refrigerator for 5 weeks in shell, and 1 week if hard-boiled.
  - Fruits and vegetables: Refrigerate perishable fruits and vegetables at 40° F (4° C). All pre-cut and pre-peeled fruits and vegetables should also be refrigerated.
  - Do not leave perishables at room temperature for more than 2 hr (1 hr if the temperature is 90° F [32° C] or above).
  - Canned goods: Check for rusting, crushing, and denting. Observe for stickiness on the outside of can, which may indicate leakage. Do not use any canned foods that are damaged.
- Foodborne illnesses
  - Salmonella: Occurs due to eating undercooked or raw meat, poultry, eggs, fish, fruit, and dairy products. Common manifestations include headache, fever, abdominal cramping, diarrhea, nausea, and vomiting. This condition can be fatal.
  - *Escherichia coli* 0157:H7: Raw or undercooked meat, especially ground beef, can cause this foodborne pathogen. Findings include severe abdominal pain and diarrhea.
  - *Listeria monocytogenes*: Soft cheese, raw milk products, undercooked poultry, processed meats, and raw vegetables can cause the illness. *Listeria monocytogenes* causes significant problems for newborns, pregnant clients, and immunocompromised clients. Onset occurs with the development of a sudden fever, diarrhea, headache, back pain, and abdominal discomfort. It can lead to stillbirth or miscarriage.
  - Norovirus: A viral infection caused by consuming contaminated fruits and vegetables, salads prepared by someone who is infected, oysters, and contaminated water. Norovirus is very contagious, and has an onset of 24 to 48 hr. Manifestations include projectile vomiting, fever, myalgia, watery diarrhea, and headache.

Ⓝ *NCLEX® Connection: Health Promotion and Maintenance, Health Promotion/Disease Prevention*

CHAPTER 6

UNIT 1   PRINCIPLES OF NUTRITION

CHAPTER 6 *Cultural, Ethnic, and Religious Influences*

Cultural, ethnic, and religious considerations greatly affect nutritional health. Understanding that ideas regarding food choices and nutrition vary among cultures prevents ethnocentrism. Identifying and incorporating individual preferences promotes client-centered care. Q︎PCC

Cultural traditions affect food choices and routines. Nurses should take this into consideration when planning and communicating nutritional goals with clients.

Acculturation is the process of a cultural, ethnic, or religious group's adopting of the dominant culture's behaviors, beliefs, and values.

Considering the client's foodway can be a helpful way to determine dietary preferences, which includes the role of foods, food preparation, what foods are considered edible, timing of meals, and use of food for health or other benefits.

CULTURE AND NUTRITION

- Culture influences every aspect of life, including nutritional intake. While common preferences exist within some cultures, individual preferences and the degree to which the client follows cultural recommendations can vary greatly. For further information on culture, refer to **FUNDAMENTALS CHAPTER 35: CULTURAL AND SPIRITUAL NURSING CARE.**
- Food might be **symbolic** for a client.
  - Representing masculinity or femininity
  - Viewed as expressions of love or punishment
  - Representing connectedness or separateness
  - Part of celebration or mourning
  - "Comfort foods" that relate to a client's past
- Culture defines what foods are **edible**, or allowable, in the diet. This idea is not always based on the nutritional value, or the visual appeal. Considerations include:
  - Whether the food is perceived as harmful
  - What foods are for animal consumption (not human)
  - Whether others within the culture consume it

- The types of foods within a culture fall into three categories regarding the **role** they have in the diet.
  - Core foods make up the majority of dietary intake (the foods eaten most often and consistently).
  - Secondary foods are not consumed as often as core foods, but are included often.
  - Peripheral foods are consumed occasionally due to cost or availability. Peripheral foods might be reserved for special days, or consumed less often because they are not well-tolerated.
- Food preparation guidelines can include how the food is obtained or prepared prior to being obtained by the client, methods of cooking, and the use of seasonings.
- The timing and frequency of meals can vary across cultures.
- Foods are often linked to health beliefs, with cultures defining what foods are helpful or not, whether or not foods are curative, and under what conditions the foods should be consumed.
  - American culture values eating foods from food groups (fruits and vegetables, grains, proteins).
  - Many cultures (Chinese, Middle Eastern, Latin American, Indian, Filipino) have health beliefs regarding hot and cold balance.
- Through acculturation, individuals and groups change their practices to reflect the dominant culture. First-generation members of a family are more likely to follow their traditional foodway, with subsequent generations incorporating the dominant culture's food practices through socialization. Acculturation of the diet can include removing or replacing traditional foods with new ones, and adding new foods to the diet.
- Dietary changes resulting from acculturation can be:
  - Positive, if the client includes more healthy foods.
  - Negative, if intake of high-fat, high-calorie, or high-sodium foods increases.

SELECTED POPULATIONS

Hispanic/Latinx

This is the predominant minority group in the U.S., with the largest percentage clients being of Mexican heritage. Certain foods are considered hot or cold and can be used to provide balance for healing. Cinnamon and teas (mint, chamomile) can be used as part of healing.

NUTRITION-RELATED CONCERNS
- High intake of fruit, dark green and orange vegetables, legumes
- Increased intake of saturated fat and sodium
- Decreased intake of whole grains and milk
- High prevalence of obesity
- Diabetes mellitus type 2 as a leading cause of death

African American

This is the second largest minority group in the U.S. Most individuals can identify a West African heritage or ancestors who immigrated through the Caribbean, Central America, or Eastern Africa. Food habits of African American clients are related more to personal factors (work schedule, location, socioeconomic status) than heritage. African Americans are more likely than white Americans accept a larger body size as normal.

NUTRITION-RELATED CONCERNS
- Score just under the national average on USDA healthy eating scores (total and saturated fat, sodium, cholesterol intake)
- Lower intake of whole grains, milk, and vegetables than clients who are white, who have a higher intake of sodium and saturated fat.
- Highest prevalence rates of obesity.
- Increased rates of diabetes mellitus with increased risk of complications
- Increased risk for hypertension, usually uncontrolled

Asian American

This is the third largest minority group in the U.S., and includes 37 different ethnic groups. The Chinese population is the largest subgroup of Asian American people. Common food patterns among this diverse group include devoting considerable skill and time to food preparation and consumption of rice and vegetables more than meats.

Many Asian cultures believe in the balance of yin and yang forces, and that, when food is digested, it turns into one of these components. Diseases associated with yin forces are treated by consuming yang foods, and yang illness with yin foods.

Yang foods: Fried foods, coffee, spice, meat, meat broths

Yin foods: Seaweed, many fruits and vegetables, cold beverages

NUTRITION-RELATED CONCERNS
- Lowest prevalence of obesity
- Highest life expectancy (Asian American females)
- Higher risk of diabetes mellitus type 2 when body fat increases (compared to other groups)

SELECTED CULTURAL DIETS

These diets common to the major subcultural groups in the United States can vary from client to client. Acculturation causes a moving away from the traditional foods in place of others.

American

- Many foods from various cultures are components of American cuisine.
- Foods are often prepared quickly or are expected to be made fast. Foods prepared at home often include premade ingredients or packaged kits to reduce mealtime preparation.

NUTRITIONAL HEALTH RISKS
- Convenience foods for home cooking are high in sodium and calories, while low in fiber.
- Portion sizes on packaged meal kits are often small, leading to consuming more than one serving.
- Meals and snacks eaten away from home are low in fruit, vegetables, dairy, and whole grains, but high in fat, sugar, and sodium.

Soul food

The soul food diet had its origins in Southern and Western Africa. Many Americans have adopted soul food practices, particularly in the Southern U.S. It is more common in low socioeconomic or rural areas.

TRADITIONAL FOODS: Rice, grits, cornbread, hominy, okra, greens, sweet potatoes, apples, peaches, buttermilk, pudding, cheddar or American cheese, ham, pork, chicken, catfish, black-eyed peas, red and pinto beans, peanuts, soft drinks, fatback

ACCULTURATION
- Buying convenience foods rather than preparing home made (breads, luncheon meat, cured meats)
- Increased milk consumption
- Possible reduced intake of fruits and vegetables if not readily available

NUTRITIONAL HEALTH RISKS
- High in fat, protein, and sodium
- Low in potassium, calcium, and fiber (protective nutrients)
- Many foods are fried

Mexican

Spanish and Native American cultures have influenced the traditional Mexican diet.

TRADITIONAL FOODS: Rice, corn, tortillas, tropical fruits, vegetables, nuts, legumes, eggs, cheese, seafood, poultry, infrequent sweets and red meat
- Tortillas eaten at most meals
- Animal protein from ground poultry, pork, goat
- Vegetables often incorporated into the main dish

ACCULTURATION
- Decreased intake of vegetables
- Intake of corn-based products replaced with flour-based
- Increased milk intake or replaced with low-fat options
- Red meat intake increased while legume intake decreased
- Increased use of fats (butter, margarine, salad dressing)
- Increased use of high-sugar, low-nutrient beverages (e.g., replacing fruit juice with carbonated sodas)

Chinese

Largest Asian American subgroup

TRADITIONAL FOODS: Wheat (northern), rice (southern), noodles, fruits, land and sea vegetables, nuts/seeds, soy foods (tofu), nut/seed oils, fish, shellfish, poultry, eggs, sweets, rarely red meats, seafoods, tea, beer
- Tofu, soups made from bone, and fish containing small bones provide most of calcium intake.

- Increased intake of wheat-based foods
- Increased intake of raw vegetables and replacement of traditional vegetables
- Increased fruit intake
- Increased intake of dairy, meat, ethnic dishes, and fast food

NUTRITIONAL-RELATED HEALTH RISKS
- Most foods are cooked, with exception of occasional fresh fruit.
- Risk of increased sodium is possible due to salting/drying to preserve foods and use of salt-based condiments.

Vegetarian diets

Semi-vegetarian/flexitarian diets are mainly plant-based diet with occasional intake of meat, poultry, dairy, or fish.

Vegetarian
- A vegetarian diet typically omits meat, seafood, poultry, or fish.
- Some clients include eggs, dairy products, fish, and/or occasional other animal products.

Vegan
- Pure vegan diets do not include animal products of any type, including eggs and milk products.
- A pure vegan diet requires a variety of plant materials to be consumed in specific combinations in order to ensure essential amino acid intake.
  - The vegan diet is adequate in protein with sufficient intake of nuts and legumes (dried peas, cooked beans).
  - Clients following a vegan diet should ensure adequate intake of iron, zinc, calcium, vitamin D, omega-3 fatty acids and vitamin B_{12}, because there is a risk of deficiency of these nutrients depending on the types of foods selected.
- A **raw vegan** diet is based on consuming uncooked plant-based foods.
- A **macrobiotic** diet is a whole-foods diet based on locally grown plants with occasional fish or seafood.

NUTRITIONAL-RELATED HEALTH RISKS: Risk for deficiency in vitamin B_{12}, vitamin D, iron, calcium, and zinc, unless the client incorporates these foods regularly.

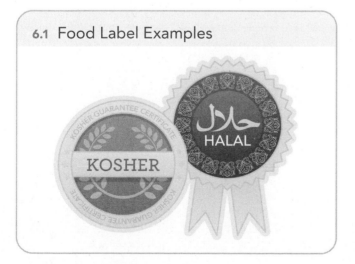

6.1 Food Label Examples

KOSHER

حلال HALAL

RELIGION AND NUTRITION

- Religion has a profound influence on foodways, especially because religion crosses geographic boundaries. Although culture and religion are linked, religion often has more of an influence on dietary practices than culture. Variations among individual denominations of a religion can vary greatly.
  - The dietary laws for Orthodox Judaism are outlined in the Torah.
  - Two Protestant Christian faiths prescribe dietary laws (Church of Jesus Christ of Latter-Day Saints [Mormon], Seventh-Day Adventists).
  - The Qur'an contains food laws for the Islamic faith. Foods are either permitted (*halal*) or prohibited (*haram*).
  - Hindu and Buddhist religions have values related to not harming living creatures (*ahimsa*), which lends to followers practicing vegetarianism.
- Some followers of a particular religion follow the moral laws but not dietary prescriptions. Always ask clients to describe their dietary preferences.

Variations based on religion

Eating on Holy Days: Some religions observe feasts on specific days (Eastern Orthodox Christian, Judaism). During Passover, Judaism calls for consumption of unleavened bread only.

Fasting for religious holidays: Islam calls for fasting during Ramadan. Roman Catholicism calls for refraining from meat consumption on Ash Wednesday and Fridays during Lent, and to avoid food or beverage intake for 1 hr before communion. Seventh-Day Adventism recommends a 5- to 6-hr interval between meals. Judaism calls for a 24-hr fast during Yom Kippur.

Restricting specific substances
- Alcohol (Islam, Hindu, Mormon, Seventh-Day Adventism)
- Pork (Seventh-Day Adventism, Orthodox Judaism, Islam, Hindu, Buddhism)
- Coffee or tea (Seventh-Day Adventism, Mormonism)
- Other: Clients who follow Orthodox Judaism might not eat meat and dairy products at the same time; *pareve* foods contain neither and can be consumed at any time. Clients who follow Judaism might consume only fish that have scales and fins.

Consuming animal products
- Vegetarian diet: Seventh-Day Adventism, Hinduism, Buddhism
- Orthodox Judaism and Islam call for consumption of Kosher animals. Both have regulations for how animals are slaughtered, particularly so that no blood is consumed.

Preparing foods: Orthodox Judaism prohibits food preparation on the Sabbath.

NURSING INTERVENTIONS

- Obtaining the client's preferences related to nutrition is vital. The information on cultural and religious influences on nutrition is so vast that the nurse should focus more on the needs of the individual clients for whom the nurse is assigned care. Ask questions regarding the following.
  - What portions of the client's diet are influenced by personal values
  - What the client considers healthy versus unhealthy
  - What food and eating means to the client
  - When the client eats meals, and if there is a sequence to the foods eaten
  - Who shops for and prepares the foods the client consumes
  - Whether the client abstains from any foods
  - Whether there are restrictions related to foods and food preparation
  - Whether foods are linked to religious practice or spiritual beliefs
  - Whether the client's beliefs dictate fasting, feasting, or types of foods consumed on specific days or dates
- Seek further information about the client's preferred dietary practices from reputable sources, as needed, to guide nutritional counseling.
- If specific foods associated with the client's culture are deemed negative medically, ask the client to reduce consumption of the foods rather than eliminating them (reducing portion size, eating less often).
- Suggest fruits and vegetables that are similar in taste or texture to what the client prefers, to increase or ensure adequate consumption.
- Seek the assistance of a dietitian to ensure the client will receive essential nutrients and to help combine medical recommendations with personal preferences.

Active Learning Scenario

A nurse is providing teaching to a group of clients who consume a primarily Mexican diet. What cultural considerations should guide the nurse with the teaching? Use the ATI Active Learning Template: Basic Concept to complete this item to include the following.

RELATED CONTENT

- Traditional foods: Include at least six foods common to this diet.
- Acculturation: Describe three examples of how food practices change as clients who follow this diet acculturate to the dominant American culture.

Application Exercises

1. A nurse is assisting a client with selecting food choices on a menu. Which of the following actions by the nurse demonstrates ethnocentrism?
   - A. Asking the client about some favorite food choices
   - B. Notifying the dietitian to complete the menu
   - C. Recommending one's own favorite foods
   - D. Asking the client's family to fill out the menu

2. A nurse is caring for a client who has hypertension. Which of the dietary patterns is sometimes followed by Asian clients and places clients at risk for this condition?
   - A. Incorporation of plant-based foods in the diet
   - B. Consumption of raw fruits
   - C. Preparation of foods using sodium
   - D. Focus on shellfish in the diet

3. A nurse educator is teaching a class on culture and food to a group of newly hired nurses. Which of the following statements by a nurse indicates an understanding of the teaching?
   - A. "Most clients who practice Roman Catholicism do not drink caffeinated beverages."
   - B. "Most clients who practice orthodox Judaism do not eat meat with dairy products."
   - C. "Most clients who are Mormon eat only the protein of animals that are slaughtered under strict guidelines."
   - D. "Most clients who practice Hinduism do not eat dairy products."

4. A nurse is reviewing the effect of culture on nutrition during a staff in-service. Which of the following groups prescribes eating specific foods to balance forces in the body during illness? (Select all that apply.)
   - A. Asian culture
   - B. African culture
   - C. Roman Catholicism
   - D. Hispanic/Latinx culture
   - E. Buddhism

Application Exercises Key

1. A. Asking the client about some favorite foods choices demonstrates sensitivity to the client's food preferences.
   B. Calling the dietitian to fill out the menu does not demonstrate sensitivity to the client's food preferences. However, it is not an example of an ethnocentric approach.
   C. **CORRECT:** Recommending one's own favorite foods is an example of ethnocentrism, which is the belief that one's own cultural practices are the only correct behaviors/beliefs.
   D. Having the family fill out the menu does not demonstrate sensitivity to the client's food preferences. However, it is not an example of an ethnocentric approach.

   Ⓝ *NCLEX® Connection: Psychosocial Integrity, Cultural Awareness/Cultural Influences on Health*

2. A. Encourage plant-based foods to increase nutrients in the diet.
   B. Encourage raw fruits in the client's diet to increase vitamin intake.
   C. **CORRECT:** The preparation of foods using sodium places the client at risk for hypertension. Many spices in the Asian diet contain sodium, or it is used as a preservative. The client should reduce sodium consumption.
   D. Encourage the consumption of shellfish because it is a good source of protein and vitamins.

   Ⓝ *NCLEX® Connection: Health Promotion and Maintenance, High Risk Behaviors*

3. A. This is generally not a practice of Roman Catholics. Caffeinated beverages are often not consumed by Mormons and Muslims because caffeine is a stimulant.
   B. **CORRECT:** Most clients who practice Orthodox Judaism do not eat meat with dairy products.
   C. Most clients who follow the teachings of Islam eat only the protein of animals that are slaughtered under strict guidelines.
   D. Most clients who practice Hinduism believe dairy products enhance spiritual purity.

   Ⓝ *NCLEX® Connection: Health Promotion and Maintenance, High Risk Behaviors*

4. A. **CORRECT:** Asian traditions can include balancing yin and yang forces within the body, and foods are grouped into those categories.
   B. African culture has influenced development of the soul food diet, but individual preferences differ widely.
   C. Roman Catholicism includes few laws related to fasting on holidays or from certain foods.
   D. **CORRECT:** Hispanic/Latinx cultural traditions can include balancing hot and cold forces within the body, and foods are grouped into those categories.
   E. Buddhism has recommendations for eating foods in a manner that do not cause harm.

   Ⓝ *NCLEX® Connection: Psychosocial Integrity, Cultural Awareness/Cultural Influences on Health*

Active Learning Scenario Key

Using the ATI Active Learning Template: Basic Concept

RELATED CONTENT
- Traditional foods
  - Grains: rice, corn
  - Tropical fruits and vegetables
  - Protein: nuts, legumes, eggs, cheese, seafood, poultry
- Acculturation
  - Increased milk use
  - Decreased vegetable consumption
  - Replacement of corn by wheat in tortillas and breads
  - Decreased bean use and change in rice preparation to plain boiled rice
  - Added fats in the form of butter or salad dressings on cooked vegetables and side salads
  - Replacement of fruit-based drinks by sugar-laden drinks

Ⓝ *NCLEX® Connection: Psychosocial Integrity, Cultural Awareness/ Cultural Influences on Health*

UNIT 1   PRINCIPLES OF NUTRITION

CHAPTER 7
Nutrition Across the Lifespan

Nutritional needs change as clients pass through the stages of the lifespan, reflecting physiological changes.

Nurses must address nutritional needs across the lifespan and have a thorough understanding of how needs change. This includes planning and implementing dietary plans that meet clients' specific needs and assist in health promotion.

Major stages of the lifespan that have specific nutritional needs include pregnancy and lactation, infancy, childhood, adolescence, and adulthood and older adulthood. Ⓖ

Pregnancy and lactation

- Prepregnancy nutrition is highly significant and plays an important role, because early fetal development occurs before a client might realize they are pregnant. A client should be well-nourished and within the normal weight range prior to conception. Low levels of folate prior to conception increases the likelihood of neural tube defects.
- Good nutrition during pregnancy is essential for the health of the unborn child.
- Maternal nutritional demands are increased for the development of the placenta, enlargement of the uterus, formation of amniotic fluid, increase in blood volume, and preparation of the breasts for lactation.
- A daily increase of 340 calories is recommended during the second trimester of pregnancy, and an increase of 452 calories is recommended during the third trimester of pregnancy.
- The nutritional requirements of clients who are pregnant or lactating involves more than increased caloric intake. Specific dietary requirements for major nutrients and micronutrients should be met.

DIETARY GUIDELINES

- Achieving an appropriate amount of weight gain during pregnancy prepares a client for the energy demands of labor and lactation, and contributes to the delivery of a newborn of normal birth weight.
- The recommended weight gain during pregnancy varies for each client depending on their body mass index (BMI) and weight prior to pregnancy. (7.1)
- Lactating clients require an increase in daily caloric intake. If the client is breastfeeding during the postpartum period, an additional daily intake of 330 calories is recommended during the first 6 months, and an additional daily intake of 400 calories is recommended during the second 6 months.

MAJOR AND MICRONUTRIENT REQUIREMENTS

- Dietary requirements for major nutrients
  - Protein should comprise 20% of the daily total calorie intake. The Dietary Reference Intake (DRI) for protein during pregnancy is 71 g/day. Protein is essential for rapid tissue growth of maternal and fetal structures, amniotic fluid, and extra blood volume. Clients who are pregnant should be aware that animal sources of protein might contain large amounts of fats.
  - Fat should be limited to 30% of total daily calorie intake.
  - Carbohydrates should comprise 50% of the total daily calorie intake. Ensuring adequate carbohydrate intake allows for protein to be spared and available for the synthesis of fetal tissue.
- The need for most vitamins and minerals increases during pregnancy and lactation. Vitamins are essential for blood formation, absorption of iron, and development of fetal tissue. TABLE 7.2 lists the comparative DRIs of major vitamins for clients age 19 to 30 during nonpregnancy, pregnancy, and lactation.

7.1 Recommended weight gain during pregnancy

FIRST TRIMESTER: Recommended weight gain is 1.1 to 4.4 lb.

SECOND AND THIRD TRIMESTERS: Recommended weight gain is 2 to 4 lb/month.
- **Normal weight client (BMI 18.5–24.9):** 1 lb/week for a total of 25 to 35 lb.
- **Underweight client (BMI < 18.5):** just more than 1 lb/week for a total of 28 to 40 lb.
- **Overweight client (BMI 25–29.9):** 0.66 lb/week for a total of 15 to 25 lb.
- **Obese client (BMI > 30):** 0.5 lb/week for a total of 11 to 20 lb.

ADDITIONAL DIETARY RECOMMENDATIONS

Fluid: 2,000 to 3,000 mL fluids daily from food and drinks. Preferred fluids include water, fruit juice, and milk. Carbonated beverages and fruit drinks provide little or no nutrients.

Alcohol: It is recommended that clients abstain from alcohol consumption during pregnancy. There is no safe recommendation for alcohol use during pregnancy.

Caffeine: Caffeine crosses the placenta and can affect the movement and heart rate of the fetus. However, moderate use (less than 200 mg/day) does not appear to be harmful.

Vegetarian diets: Well-balanced vegetarian diets that include dairy products can provide all the nutritional requirements of pregnancy.

Folic acid intake: It is recommended that 600 mcg/day of folic acid be taken during pregnancy. Current recommendations for lactating clients include 500 mcg/day folic acid. It is necessary for the neurologic development of the fetus and to prevent birth defects. It is essential for maternal red blood cell formation. Clients who have had a child born with a neural tube defect should consume 4 mg daily of folic acid during pregnancy. Food sources include green leafy vegetables, enriched grains, and orange juice.
- Folic acid is the synthetic form of folate and is absorbed better by the body. Folic acid is found in supplements and in fortified foods.
- Folate is found in natural foods.

Iron: The DRI for iron increases by 50% during pregnancy to support the increase in maternal blood volume and to provide iron for fetal liver storage. Iron can be obtained from meats, eggs, leafy greens, enriched breads, and dried fruits. Consuming foods high in vitamin C aids in the absorption of iron. It is recommended that pregnant clients take a supplement of 27 to 30 mg iron daily to assure adequate intake.

Nonnutritive sweeteners: Several nonnutritive sweeteners have been approved for use during pregnancy. Occasional use is not considered harmful, but it is not known if they are beneficial.

Fish: The FDA has issued advisories regarding fish and shellfish consumption during pregnancy due to the risk of mercury levels. Mercury can be toxic to developing fetal brain tissue. Fish are a good source of omega 3 fatty acids, which are important for fetal brain and eye development.
- Limit albacore tuna to 6 oz/week.
- Avoid tilefish, shark, swordfish, marlin, orange roughy, and king mackerel due to mercury content.
- Limit weekly consumption of seafood to 12 oz.

DIETARY COMPLICATIONS

Nausea and constipation are common during pregnancy.
- For nausea, eat dry crackers, toast, and salty or tart foods. Avoid alcohol, caffeine, fats, and spices. Avoid drinking fluids with meals, and do not take medications to control nausea without checking with the provider.
- For constipation, increase fluid consumption (at least 8 cups per day) and include extra fiber in the diet. Fruits, vegetables, and whole grains contain fiber.
- Regular physical activity can minimize or prevent constipation.

Maternal phenylketonuria (PKU) is a maternal genetic disease in which high levels of phenylalanine pose danger to the fetus.
- It is important for a client to start the PKU diet at least 3 months prior to pregnancy, and continue the diet throughout pregnancy.
- The diet should include foods low in phenylalanine. Foods high in protein (fish, poultry, meat, eggs, nuts, dairy products) must be avoided due to high phenylalanine levels. Qs
- The client's blood phenylalanine levels should be monitored during pregnancy.
- These interventions will prevent fetal complications (intellectual disability, behavioral problems).

ASSESSMENT/DATA COLLECTION AND INTERVENTIONS

- Nursing assessments should include a complete profile of the client's knowledge base regarding nutritional requirements during pregnancy.
- Nurses should review with the client the recommended dietary practices for pregnant and lactating clients, while providing materials containing this information.

7.2 DRIs of major vitamins

NUTRIENT	NONPREGNANT	PREGNANT	LACTATING
Protein	46 g	71 g	71 g
Vitamin A	700 mcg	770 mcg	1,300 mcg
Vitamin C	75 mg	85 mg	120 mg
Vitamin D*	15 mcg	15 mcg	15 mcg
Vitamin E	15 mcg	15 mcg	19 mcg
Vitamin K*	90 mcg	90 mcg	90 mcg
Thiamin	1.1 mg	1.4 mg	1.4 mg
Vitamin B$_6$	1.3 mg	1.9 mg	2.0 mg
Folic acid	400 mcg	600 mcg	500 mcg
Vitamin B$_{12}$	2.4 mcg	2.6 mcg	2.8 mcg
Calcium*	1,000 mg	1,000 mg	1,000 mg
Iron	18 mg	27 mg	9 mg

*Values represent adequate intakes.

Source: Office of Dietary Supplements. National Institutes of Health, ods.od.nih.gov

Infancy

- Growth rate during infancy is more rapid than any other period of the life cycle. It is important to understand normal growth patterns to determine the adequacy of an infant's nutritional intake.
- Birth weight doubles by 4 to 6 months and triples by 1 year of age. The need for calories and nutrients is high to support the rapid rate of growth.
- Appropriate weight gain averages 0.15 to 0.21 kg (5 to 7 oz) per week during the first 5 to 6 months.
- An infant grows approximately 2.5 cm (1 in) per month in height during the first 6 months, and approximately 1.25 cm (0.5 in) per month during the second 6 months.
- Head circumference increases rapidly during the first 6 months at a rate of 1.5 cm (0.6 in) per month. The rate slows to 0.5 cm/month for months 6 to 12. By 1 year, head size should have increased by 33%. This is reflective of the growth of the nervous system.
- Breast milk, infant formula, or a combination of the two is the sole source of nutrition for the first 6 months of life.
- Semisolid foods should not be introduced before 6 months of age to coincide with the development of the gastrointestinal system, head control, ability to sit, and the back-and-forth motion of the tongue.
- Gestational iron stores begin to deplete around 4 months of age, so iron supplementation is recommended after this time for infants who are exclusively fed breast milk. Once solid foods are introduced, iron-fortified cereal is a good source of iron.
- Cow's milk should not be introduced into the diet until after 1 year of age because protein and mineral content stress the immature kidney. A young infant cannot fully digest the protein and fat contained in cow's milk.

MEETING NUTRITIONAL NEEDS

Additional information about feeding is available in **MATERNAL NEWBORN CHAPTER 25: NEWBORN NUTRITION** and **NURSING CARE OF CHILDREN CHAPTER 3 : HEALTH PROMOTION OF INFANTS (2 DAYS TO 1 YEAR).**

BREASTFEEDING

- The American Academy of Pediatrics (AAP), World Health Organization (WHO), Department of Health and Human Services (HHS), and American College of Obstetricians and Gynecologists recommend that infants receive breast milk for the first 6 to 12 months of age (exclusive breast feeding) followed by breastfeeding with the introduction of complementary foods until at least 12 months of age, then continuation of breastfeeding for as long as the parent and infant desire. Even a short period of breastfeeding has physiological benefits.

- Donor milk can be considered in certain circumstances.
  - The choice to feed an infant human milk from a source other than the infant's parent should be made in consultation with the provider, because the nutritional needs of each infant depend on many factors, including the infant's age and health.
  - The FDA recommends that if an infant is to be fed human milk from a source other than the infant's parent, use only milk from a source that has screened its donors and take other precautions to ensure the safety of the milk. Qs
- The AAP recommends that for the first 6 months, infants should receive no water or formula except in cases of medical indication or informed parental choice. In the hospital, no water or formula should be given to a breastfed infant unless prescribed by a provider. QEBP

Nutritional advantages of breast milk

- Carbohydrates, proteins, and fats in breast milk are predigested for ready absorption.
- Breast milk is high in omega-3 fatty acids.
- Breast milk is low in sodium.
- Iron, zinc, and magnesium found in breast milk are highly absorbable.
- Calcium absorption is enhanced, as the calcium-to-phosphorous ratio is 2:1.

Breastfeeding teaching points

- The newborn is offered the breast immediately after birth and frequently thereafter. There should be eight to 12 feedings in a 24-hr period.
- Instruct the client to demand-feed the infant and to assess for hunger cues. These include rooting, suckling on hands and fingers, and rapid eye movement. Crying is a late indicator of hunger.
- The newborn should nurse up to 15 min per breast. Findings that indicate the newborn has completed the feeding include the slowing of newborn suckling, a softened breast, or sleeping. Eventually, the infant will empty a breast within 5 to 10 min, but might need to continue to suck to meet comfort needs. QEBP
- Do not offer the newborn any supplements unless indicated by the provider.
- Frequent feedings (every 2 hr can be indicated) and manual expression of milk to initiate flow can be needed.
- Awaken the infant to feed every 3 hr during the day and every 4 hr at night.
- Encourage clients to express breast milk for supplementation if extra fluids or calories are required.
- Expressed milk can be refrigerated in sterile bottles or storage bags and labeled with the date and time the milk was expressed. It can be maintained in the refrigerator for 24 hr or frozen in sterile containers for 3 months.
- Thaw milk in the refrigerator. It can be stored for 24 hr after thawing. Defrosting or heating in a microwave oven is not recommended because high heat destroys some of milk's antibodies, and can burn the infant's oral mucosa.

- Do not refreeze thawed milk.
- Unused breast milk must be discarded.
- Limit alcohol and caffeine while breastfeeding.
- Begin manual expression of the breast or use an electric breast pump if the infant is unable to breastfeed due to prematurity or respiratory distress.

FORMULA FEEDING

Can be used in place of breastfeeding, as an occasional supplement to breastfeeding, or when exclusively breastfed infants are weaned before 12 months of age.

- Commercial infant formulas provide an alternative to breast milk. They are modified from cow's milk to provide comparable nutrients. However, breast milk is superior to any formula and even more crucial for a premature infant.
- If formula-fed, an iron-fortified formula is recommended for at least the first 12 months of life or until the infant consumes adequate solid food.
- Fluoride supplements can be required if an adequate level is not supplied by the water supply.
- Precisely follow the manufacturer's mixing directions.
- Bottles of mixed formula or open cans of liquid formula require refrigeration. Do not use if the formula has been left at room temperature for 2 hr or longer. Do not reuse partially emptied bottles of formula.
- Formula can be fed chilled, warmed, or at room temperature. Always give formula at approximately the same temperature.
- The infant should not drink more than 32 oz formula per 24 hr period unless directed by a provider.

BOTTLE FEEDING

- Hold the infant during feedings with the head slightly elevated to facilitate passage of formula or breast milk into the stomach. Tilt the bottle to maintain liquid in the nipple and prevent the swallowing of air.
- Do not prop the bottle or put an infant to bed with a bottle. This practice promotes tooth decay.

INTRODUCING SOLID FOOD

- Indicators for readiness include voluntary control of the head and trunk, hunger less than 4 hr after vigorous nursing or intake of 8 oz of formula, and interest of the infant.
- New foods should be introduced one at a time over a 5- to 7-day period to observe for indications of allergy or intolerance, which can include fussiness, rash, upper respiratory distress, vomiting, diarrhea, or constipation. The order of introduction of new foods is no longer considered important, and meat can be introduced first due to its iron and zinc content. ○EBP
- The infant can be ready for three meals per day with three snacks by 8 months of age.
- Homemade baby food is an acceptable feeding option. Do not use canned or packaged foods that are high in sodium. Select fresh or frozen foods, and do not add sugars or other seasonings.

- Open jars of infant food can be stored in the refrigerator for up to 24 hr.
- By 9 months of age, the infant should be able to eat table foods that are cooked, chopped, and unseasoned.
- Do not feed the infant honey due to the risk of botulism.
- Appropriate finger foods include ripe bananas, toast strips, graham crackers, cheese cubes, noodles, and peeled chunks of apples, pears, or peaches.

NUTRITION-RELATED PROBLEMS

Colic

Colic is characterized by persistent crying lasting 3 hr or longer per day.

- The cause of colic is unknown, but usually occurs in the late afternoon, more than 3 days per week for more than 3 weeks. The crying is accompanied by a tense abdomen and legs drawn up to the belly.
- If breastfeeding, eliminate cruciferous vegetables (cauliflower, broccoli, and Brussels sprouts), cow's milk, onion, and chocolate, and limit caffeine and nicotine.
- Burp the infant in an upright position.

Lactose intolerance

Lactose intolerance is the inability to digest significant amounts of lactose (the predominant sugar of milk) and is due to inadequate lactase (the enzyme that digests lactose into glucose and galactose).

- Lactose intolerance has an increased prevalence in individuals of Asian, Native American, African, Latino, and Mediterranean descent.
- Findings include abdominal distention, flatus, and occasional diarrhea.
- Soy-based or casein hydrolysate formulas can be prescribed as alternative formulas for infants who are lactose intolerant.

Failure to thrive

Failure to thrive is defined as inadequate gains in weight and height in comparison to established growth and development norms (weight-for-length less than 5th percentile or weight for age below the 3rd percentile).

- Assess for findings of congenital defects, central nervous system disorders, or partial intestinal obstruction.
- Monitor for swallowing or sucking problems.
- Identify feeding patterns, especially concerning preparation of formulas.
- Observe for psychosocial problems, especially impaired caregiver–infant bonding, abuse/neglect.
- Provide supportive nutritional guidance. Usually a high-calorie, high-protein diet is indicated.
- Provide supportive parenting guidance.

Diarrhea

Diarrhea is characterized by the passage of more than three loose, watery stools over a 24-hr period.

- Overfeeding and food intolerances are common causes of osmotic diarrhea.
- Infectious diarrhea in the infant is commonly caused by rotavirus.
- Mild diarrhea can require no specific interventions. Check with the provider for any diet modifications.
- Treatment for moderate diarrhea should begin at home with oral rehydration solutions. After each loose stool, an 8 oz solution should be given. Sports drinks are contraindicated.
- Educate parents about the findings of dehydration: listlessness, sunken eyes, sunken fontanels, decreased tears, dry mucous membranes, and decreased urine output.
- Breastfed infants should continue nursing.
- Formula-fed infants usually do not require diluted formulas or special formulas.
- Contact the provider if findings of dehydration are present, or if vomiting, bloody stools, high fever, change in mental status, or refusal to take liquids occurs.

Constipation

Constipation is the inability or difficulty to evacuate the bowels.

- Constipation is not a common problem for breastfed infants.
- Constipation can be caused by formula that is too concentrated.
- Stress the importance of accurate dilution of formula.
- Advise adherence to the recommended amount of formula intake for age.

NURSING ASSESSMENT/DATA COLLECTION AND INTERVENTIONS

- Nursing assessments should include an assessment of knowledge base of the client regarding nutritional guidelines for infants, normal infant growth patterns, breastfeeding, formula feeding, and the progression for the introduction of solid foods.
- Additionally, nurses should provide education and references for the client regarding each of the assessments listed above.

Childhood

- Growth rate slows following infancy.
- ChooseMyPlate.gov is a food guidance system that offers an Internet-based tool to provide clients with individualized recommendations for adequate nutrition. Children require the same food groups as adults, but in smaller serving sizes. Qↄ
- Energy needs and appetite vary with the child's activity level and growth rate.
- Generally, nutrient needs increase with age.
- Attitudes toward food and general food habits are established by 5 years of age.
- Increasing the variety and texture of foods helps the child develop good eating habits.
- Foods like hot dogs, popcorn, peanuts, grapes, raw carrots, celery, peanut butter, tough meat, and candy can cause choking or aspiration. Qs
- Inclusion in family mealtime is important for social development.
- Group eating becomes a significant means of socialization for school-age children.

TODDLERS: 1 TO 3 YEARS OLD

NUTRITION GUIDELINES

- Toddlers generally grow 2 to 3 inches in height and gain approximately 5 to 6 lb/year.
- Limit 100% juice to 4 to 6 oz a day.
- The 1- to 2-year-old child requires whole cow's milk to provide adequate fat for the still-growing brain.
- Food serving size is 1 tbsp for each year of age.
- Exposure to a new food might be needed 15 to 20 times before the child develops an acceptance of it.
- If there is a negative family history for allergies, cow's milk, chocolate, citrus fruits, egg white, seafood, and nut butters can be gradually introduced while monitoring the child for reactions.
- Toddlers prefer finger foods because of their increasing autonomy. They prefer plain foods to mixtures, but usually like macaroni and cheese, spaghetti, and pizza.
- Regular meal times and nutritious snacks best meet nutrient needs.
- Snacks or desserts that are high in sugar, fat, or sodium should be avoided.
- Children are at an increased risk for choking until 4 years of age.
- Avoid foods that are potential choking hazards. Always provide adult supervision during snack and mealtimes. During food preparation, cut small, bite-sized pieces that are easy to swallow to prevent choking. Do not allow the child to engage in drinking or eating during play activities or while lying down. Qs

NUTRITIONAL CONCERNS/RISKS

Iron

- Iron deficiency anemia is the most common nutritional deficiency disorder in children.
- Lean red meats provide sources of readily absorbable iron.
- Consuming vitamin C (orange juice, tomatoes) with plant sources of iron (beans, raisins, peanut butter, whole grains) will maximize absorption.
- Milk should be limited to the recommended quantities (24 oz) because it is a poor source of iron and can displace the intake of iron-rich foods.

Vitamin D

- Vitamin D is essential for bone development.
- Recommended vitamin D intake is the same (5 mcg/day) from birth through age 50. Children require more vitamin D because their bones are growing.
- Milk (cow, soy) and fatty fish are good sources of vitamin D.
- Sunlight exposure leads to vitamin D synthesis. Children who spend large amounts of time inside (watching TV, playing video games) are at an increased risk for vitamin D deficiency.
- Vitamin D assists in the absorption of calcium into the bones.

PRESCHOOLERS: 3 TO 6 YEARS

NUTRITION GUIDELINES

- Preschoolers generally grow 2 to 3 inches in height and gain approximately 5 to 6 lb/year.
- Preschoolers need to consume 13 to 19 g/day of complete protein.
- If the preschooler consumes foods from all five food groups and height and weight are within expected reference ranges, supplemental vitamins/minerals might not be needed.
- Preschoolers tend to dislike strong-tasting vegetables (cabbage, onions), but like many raw vegetables that are eaten as finger foods.
- Food jags (ritualistic preference for one food) are common and usually short-lived.
- MyPlate guidelines are appropriate, requiring the lowest number of servings per food group.
- Food patterns and preferences are first learned from the family, and peers begin influencing preferences and habits at around 5 years of age.

NUTRITIONAL CONCERNS/RISKS

Concerns include overfeeding; intake of high-calorie, high-fat, high-sodium snacks, soft drinks, and juices; and inadequate intake of fruits and vegetables.
- Be alert to the appropriate serving size of foods (1 tbsp per year of age).
- Avoid high-fat and high-sugar snacks.
- Encourage daily physical activities.
- Can switch to skim or 1% low-fat milk after 2 years of age.

Iron deficiency anemia

Lead poisoning is a risk for children younger than 6 years of age because they frequently place objects in their mouths that can contain lead and have a higher rate of intestinal absorption.
- Feed children at frequent intervals because more lead is absorbed on an empty stomach. Qs
- Inadequate intake of calories, calcium, iron, zinc, and phosphorous can increase susceptibility.

SCHOOL-AGE CHILDREN: 6 TO 12 YEARS

NUTRITION GUIDELINES

- School-age children generally grow 2 to 3 inches in height and gain approximately 5 to 6 lb/year.
- Following MyPlate recommendations, the diet should provide variety, balance, and moderation.
- Young athletes need to meet energy, protein, and fluid needs.
- Educate children to make healthy food selections.
- Children enjoy learning how to safely prepare nutritious snacks.
- Children need to learn to eat snacks only when hungry, not when bored or inactive.

NUTRITIONAL CONCERNS/RISKS

Not eating breakfast occurs in about 10% of children.
- Optimum performance in school is dependent on a nutritious breakfast.
- Children who regularly eat breakfast tend to have an age-appropriate BMI.

Overweight/obesity affects at least 20% of children.
- Greater psychosocial implications exist for children than adults.
- Overweight children tend to be obese adults.
- Prevention is essential. Encourage healthy eating habits, decrease fats and sugars (empty-calorie foods), and increase the level of physical activity.
- A weight-loss program directed by a provider is indicated for children who are overweight, or obese if they have comorbidity. Otherwise, efforts are directed at maintaining weight so the BMI will normalize as height increases.
- Praise the child's abilities and skills.
- Never use food as a reward or punishment.

NURSING ASSESSMENT/DATA COLLECTION AND INTERVENTIONS

Nursing assessments should include the parent's knowledge base of the child's nutritional requirements, and nutritional concerns with regard to age. Nurses should provide education for the parent and child about nutritional recommendations.

Adolescence

- The rate of growth during adolescence is second only to the rate in infancy. Nutritional needs for energy, protein, calcium, iron, and zinc increase at the onset of puberty and the growth spurt.
- The female adolescent growth spurt usually begins at 10 or 11 years of age, peaks at 12 years, and is completed by 17 years. Female energy requirements are less than that of males, as they experience less growth of muscle and bone tissue and more fat deposition.
- The male adolescent growth spurt begins at 12 or 13 years of age, peaks at 14 years, and is completed by 21 years.
- Eating habits of adolescents are often inadequate in meeting recommended nutritional intake goals.

NUTRITIONAL CONSIDERATIONS

- Energy requirements average 2,000 cal/day for a 12- to 18-year-old female and 2,200 to 2,800 cal/day for a 12- to 18-year-old male.
- The USDA reports that the average U.S. adolescent consumes a diet deficient in folate, vitamins A and E, iron, zinc, magnesium, calcium, and fiber. This trend is more pronounced in females than males.
- Diets of adolescents generally exceed recommendations for total fat, saturated fat, cholesterol, sodium, and sugar.

NUTRITIONAL RISKS

Eating and snacking patterns promote essential nutrient deficiencies (calcium, vitamins, iron, fiber) and overconsumption of sugars, fat, and sodium.

- Adolescents tend to skip meals, especially breakfast, and eat more meals away from home.
- Foods are often selected from vending machines, convenience stores, and fast food restaurants. These foods are typically high in fat, sugar, and sodium.
- Carbonated beverages can replace milk and fruit juices in the diet with resulting deficiencies in vitamin C, riboflavin, phosphorous, and calcium.

Increased need for iron

- Females 14 to 18 years of age require 15 mg/day of iron to support expansion of blood volume and blood loss during menstruation.
- Males 14 to 18 years of age require 11 mg/day of iron to support expansion of muscle mass and blood volume.

Inadequate calcium intake can predispose the adolescent to osteoporosis later in life.

- During adolescence, 45% of bone mass is added.
- Normal blood-calcium levels are maintained by drawing calcium from the bones if calcium intake is low.
- Adolescents require at least 1,300 mg/day of calcium, which can be achieved by three to four servings from the dairy food group.

Dieting

- The stigma of obesity and social pressure to be thin can lead to unhealthy eating practices and poor body image, especially in females.
- Males are more susceptible to using supplements and high-protein drinks in order to build muscle mass and improve athletic performance. Some athletes restrict calories to maintain or achieve a lower weight.
- Eating disorders can follow self-imposed crash diets for weight loss.

Eating disorders (anorexia nervosa, bulimia nervosa, binge eating disorder) commonly begin during adolescence. These disorders are discussed further in the **MENTAL HEALTH REVIEW MODULE, CHAPTER 19: EATING DISORDERS**.

Adolescent pregnancy

- The physiologic demands of a growing fetus compromise the adolescent's needs for their own unfinished growth and development.
- Inconsistent eating and poor food choices place the adolescent at risk for anemia, pregnancy-induced hypertension, gestational diabetes, premature labor, miscarriage, and delivery of a newborn of low birth weight.

NURSING ASSESSMENT/DATA COLLECTION AND INTERVENTIONS

- Nursing assessments should include a determination of the following in the adolescent.
  - Typical 24-hr food intake
  - Weight patterns, current weight, and body mass index (BMI)
  - Attitude about current weight
  - Use of nutritional supplements, vitamins, and minerals
  - Medical history and use of prescription medications
  - Use of over-the-counter medications
  - Use of substances (marijuana, alcohol, tobacco)
  - Level of daily physical activity
- Assess for findings of an eating disorder. This can include an evaluation of the adolescent's laboratory values.
- Nursing assessments should include strategies that promote health for the adolescent.
  - Educate the adolescent on using MyPlate to meet energy and nutrient needs with three regular meals and snacks.
  - Stress the importance of meeting calcium needs by including low-fat milk, yogurt, and cheese in the diet.
  - Educate the adolescent on how to select and prepare nutrient-dense snack foods: unbuttered, unsalted popcorn; pretzels; fresh fruit; string cheese; smoothies made with low-fat yogurt, skim milk, or reduced-calorie fruit juice; and raw vegetables with low-fat dips. Qpcc
  - Encourage participation in vigorous physical activity at least three times per week.
  - Refer pregnant adolescents to the Women, Infant, and Children (WIC) nutrition subsidy program.
  - Provide individual and group counseling for adolescents who have findings of eating disorders.

Adulthood and older adulthood

- A balanced diet for all adults consists of 45% to 65% carbohydrates and 20% to 35% fat (with 10% or less from saturated fats).
- The recommended amount for protein is unchanged in adults and older adults. However, many nutrition experts believe that protein requirements increase in older adults.
- Older adults need to reduce total caloric intake. This is due to the decrease in basal metabolic rate that occurs from the decrease in lean body mass that develops with aging. ©
- Reduced caloric intake predisposes the older adult for development of nutrient deficiencies.
- Older adults can have physical, mental, and social changes that affect their ability to purchase, prepare, and digest foods and nutrients.
- Dehydration is the most common fluid and electrolyte imbalance in older adults. Fluid needs increase with medication-induced fluid losses. Some disease processes necessitate fluid restrictions.
- BMI should be between 18.5 and 24.9. There is an increased risk for both overweight and underweight older adult clients. Overweight adults are more prone to hypertension, diabetes mellitus, and stroke.

NUTRITIONAL CONCERNS

- A 24-hr dietary intake is helpful in determining the need for dietary education.
- Older adults can have oral problems (ill-fitting dentures, difficulty chewing or swallowing), and a decrease in salivation or poor dental health. ©
- Older adults have decreased cellular function and reduced body reserves, leading to decreased absorption of multiple vitamins and minerals as well as reductions in insulin production and sensitivity.
- Older adults have a decreased lean muscle mass. Exercise can help to counteract muscle mass loss.
- The loss of calcium can result in decreased bone density in older adults.

BALANCED DIET AND NUTRIENT NEEDS

MyPlate suggests the following daily food intake for adults and older adults who get less than 30 min of moderate physical activity most days. **(7.3)**

Grains: Select whole grains.

Vegetables: Select orange and dark green leafy vegetables.

Fruits: Select fresh, dried, canned, or juices. Avoid fruits with added sugar.

Make half your plate vegetables and fruits.

Milk, yogurt, and cheese group: One cup of milk or plain yogurt is equivalent to 1 ½ oz of natural cheese or 2 oz processed cheese.

Protein foods group: Includes meat, fish, poultry, dry beans, eggs, soy products, seeds, and nuts. One ounce–equivalent equals 1 oz meat, fish, or poultry (baked, grilled, broiled); ¼ cup cooked beans; 1 egg; 1 tbsp peanut butter; or ½ oz nuts or seeds. Use lean meats.

Oils: Use vegetable oils (except palm and coconut). One tbsp of oil equals 3 tsp equivalent; 1 tbsp equals 2 ½ tsp dietary intake; and 1 oz nuts equals 3 tsp oils (except hazelnut, which equals 4 tsp).

Discretionary calories: 132 to 362 discretionary calories are permitted per day. These add up quickly and can be from more than one food group.

Minerals: Calcium requirements increase for older adults as the efficiency of calcium absorption decreases with age.

Vitamins: Vitamins A, D, C, E, B_6, and B_{12} can be decreased in older adults. Supplemental vitamins are recommended. ©

7.3 MyPlate recommendations for adults

	MALES			FEMALES		
	19 TO 30 YEARS	31 TO 50 YEARS	51+ YEARS	19 TO 30 YEARS	31 TO 50 YEARS	51+ YEARS
Calories	2,400	2,200	2,000	2,000	1,800	1,600
Fruits	2 cups	2 cups	2 cups	2 cups	1 ½ cups	1 ½ cups
Vegetables	3 cups	3 cups	2 ½ cups	2 ½ cups	2 ½ cups	2 cups
Grains	8 oz	7 oz	6 oz	6 oz	6 oz	5 oz
Protein	6 ½ oz-eq	6 oz-eq	5 ½ oz-eq	5 ½ oz-eq	5 oz-eq	5 oz-eq
Milk	3 cups	3 cups	3 cups	3 cups	3 cups	3 cups
Oils	7 tsp	6 tsp	6 tsp	6 tsp	5 tsp	5 tsp

Source: United States Department of Agriculture. ChooseMyPlate.gov.
Retrieved December 22, 2015, from www.choosemyplate.gov

REGULAR EXERCISE

- All adults should exercise at a moderate or vigorous pace for at least 150 min per week. Adults who cannot do 150 min of moderate activity should be as physically active as tolerated.
- Moderate activities include gardening/yard work, golf, dancing, and walking briskly.
- The loss of lean muscle mass is part of normal aging and can be decreased with regular exercise. The loss of lean muscle can be associated with a decrease in total protein and insulin sensitivity.
- Regular exercise can improve bone density, relieve depression, and enhance cardiovascular and respiratory function.

POTENTIAL EFFECT OF PHYSICAL, MENTAL, AND SOCIAL CHANGES

- Diseases and treatments can interfere with nutrient and food absorption, and utilization.
  - Aging adults are at an increased risk for developing osteoporosis (decreasing total bone mass and deterioration of bone tissue). Adequate calcium and vitamin D intake with regular weight-bearing exercise is important for maximizing bone density. Ⓖ
  - Musculoskeletal concerns, such as arthritis, cause pain that can interfere with the purchase and preparation of foods.
  - Dementia can make shopping, storing, and cooking food difficult.
- Medications can cause electrolyte losses.
- Loss of smell and vision interfere with the interest in eating food.
- Older adults can have difficulty chewing, in which case mincing or chopping food is helpful. They can have difficulty swallowing food, and thickened liquids can decrease the risk for aspiration.
- Social isolation, loss of a partner, and mental deterioration can cause poor nutrition in adult and older adult clients. Encourage socialization and refer to a senior center or program. Ⓠpcc
- A fixed income can make it difficult for older adults to purchase needed foods. Refer to food programs, senior centers, and food banks. Meals on Wheels programs are available for housebound older adults.

FLUID INTAKE

- The long-held standard of consuming eight 8-oz glasses of liquid per day has been tempered by evidence that dehydration is not imminent even when less than 64 oz of fluid is consumed.
- Solid foods provide varying amounts of water, making it possible to get adequate fluid despite low beverage intake.
- For healthy adults, it is generally acceptable to allow normal drinking and eating habits to provide needed fluids.
- Encourage water and natural juices, and discourage drinking only soda pop and other liquids that have caffeine.

NURSING ASSESSMENT/DATA COLLECTION AND INTERVENTIONS

- Nursing assessments should include a dietary profile of the adult or older adult. Medical history, medication regimen, mobility, social practices, mental status, and financial circumstances are important components of the assessment.
- Nurses should provide education about dietary practices for the adult and older adult, while additionally providing referrals to registered dietitians and community agencies when needed.

Application Exercises

1. A nurse at a community center is providing nutrition counseling for a group of older adult clients. Which of the following information should the nurse include? (Select all that apply.)

   A. Increase protein to 50% of daily calories.

   B. The need for vitamins and minerals can increase.

   C. Up to 35% of daily calories should come from fat.

   D. At least 45% of daily calories should come from carbohydrates.

   E. Fruits and vegetables should make up one-third of each meal.

2. A nurse is assessing a 6-month-old infant who has a lactose intolerance. Which of the following findings should the nurse expect? (Select all that apply.)

   A. Abdominal distention

   B. Flatus

   C. Hypoactive bowel sounds

   D. Occasional diarrhea

   E. Visible peristalsis

3. A nurse is educating the parents of a toddler about appropriate snack foods. Which of the following foods should the nurse include? (Select all that apply.)

   A. Graham crackers

   B. Apple slices

   C. Raisins

   D. Jelly beans

   E. Cheese cubes

4. A nurse is teaching a group of clients who are pregnant about iron-rich foods. Which of the following foods should the nurse include? (Select all that apply.)

   A. Beans

   B. Fish

   C. Dairy products

   D. Lean red meats

   E. Apples

5. A school nurse is teaching a group of adolescents about healthy snack food choices. Which of the following foods should the nurse include? (Select all that apply.)

   A. Carrot sticks with low-fat dip

   B. Cheese and crackers

   C. Unbuttered popcorn

   D. French fries

   E. Hot dog

Active Learning Scenario

A community health nurse is teaching a group of guardians the importance of adequate vitamin D intake for children. Use the ATI Active Learning Template: Basic Concept to complete this item.

UNDERLYING PRINCIPLES

- Explain why vitamin D is important for children.
- Identify at least two sources of vitamin D.

Application Exercises Key

1. A. Protein requirements do not increase during older adulthood.
   B. **CORRECT:** Age-related changes can reduce the body's ability to absorb vitamins and minerals.
   C. **CORRECT:** Adult clients should obtain 20% to 35% of daily calories from fat.
   D. **CORRECT:** Adult clients should obtain 45% to 65% of daily calories from carbohydrates.
   E. Fruits and vegetables should make up one-half of each meal.

   Ⓝ *NCLEX® Connection: Health Promotion and Maintenance, Health Promotion/Disease Prevention*

2. A. **CORRECT:** Abdominal distention is a finding associated with a lactose intolerance.
   B. **CORRECT:** Flatus is a finding associated with a lactose intolerance.
   C. Hypoactive bowel sounds are not associated with a lactose intolerance.
   D. **CORRECT:** Occasional diarrhea is a finding associated with a lactose intolerance.
   E. Visible peristalsis is not associated with a lactose intolerance.

   Ⓝ *NCLEX® Connection: Health Promotion and Maintenance, Aging Process*

3. A. **CORRECT:** Graham crackers are appropriate snack foods for toddlers.
   B. **CORRECT:** Apple slices are appropriate snack foods for toddlers.
   C. Raisins are difficult to chew and pose a choking hazard.
   D. Jelly beans are difficult to swallow, pose a choking risk, and are high in sugar content.
   E. **CORRECT:** Cheese cubes are appropriate snack foods for toddlers.

   Ⓝ *NCLEX® Connection: Health Promotion and Maintenance, Aging Process*

4. A. **CORRECT:** Iron-rich foods include beans.
   B. **CORRECT:** Iron-rich foods include fish.
   C. Dairy products are not rich in iron.
   D. **CORRECT:** Iron-rich foods include lean red meats.
   E. Apples are not rich in iron.

   Ⓝ *NCLEX® Connection: Health Promotion and Maintenance, Ante/Intra/Postpartum and Newborn Care*

5. A. **CORRECT:** Carrot sticks with low-fat ranch dip are a healthy snack selection.
   B. **CORRECT:** Cheese and crackers are a healthy snack selection.
   C. **CORRECT:** Unbuttered popcorn is a healthy snack selection.
   D. French fries are not a healthy food choice because they are high in fat.
   E. Hot dogs are not a healthy food choice because they are high in sodium and fat.

   Ⓝ *NCLEX® Connection: Health Promotion and Maintenance, Aging Process*

Active Learning Scenario Key

Using the ATI Active Learning Template: Basic Concept

UNDERLYING PRINCIPLES
- Vitamin D is essential for the development of healthy bones. It is important in children because their bones are newly formed and continually growing.
- Vitamin D aids in the absorption of calcium into the bones. Sunlight exposure, milk (cow's, soy), and fatty fish are sources of vitamin D.

Ⓝ *NCLEX® Connection: Health Promotion and Maintenance, Aging Process*

NCLEX® Connections

When reviewing the following chapters, keep in mind the relevant topics and tasks of the NCLEX outline, in particular:

Basic Care and Comfort

NUTRITION AND ORAL HYDRATION
Manage the client's nutritional intake.

Provide client nutrition through tube feedings.

Evaluate side effects of client tube feedings and intervene, as needed.

Monitor the client's nutritional status.

Pharmacological and Parental Therapies

TOTAL PARENTERAL NUTRITION (TPN)
Administer parenteral nutrition and evaluate client response.

Apply knowledge of nursing procedures and psychomotor skills when caring for a client receiving TPN.

Reduction of Risk Potential

LABORATORY VALUES: Compare client laboratory values to normal laboratory values.

POTENTIAL FOR ALTERATIONS IN BODY SYSTEMS
Identify client potential for skin breakdown.

Identify client potential for aspiration.

UNIT 2   CLINICAL NUTRITION

CHAPTER 8 *Modified Diets*

Therapeutic nutrition is the role of food and nutrition in the treatment of diseases and disorders. The basic diet becomes therapeutic when modifications are made to meet client needs. Modifications can include increasing or decreasing caloric intake, fiber, or other specific nutrients; omitting specific foods; and modifying the consistency of foods.

It is important to remember, however, that food meets both physiological and psychological needs and should be a pleasant experience for the hospitalized client. Nurses should collaborate with the dietitian for nutritional or dietary concerns. Q**Tc**

TYPES OF MODIFIED DIETS

Regular diet (normal or house diet)

- Indicated for clients who do not need dietary restrictions. The diet is adjusted to meet age specific needs throughout the life cycle.
- Many health care facilities offer self-select menus for regular diets.
- Modify the regular diet to accommodate individual preferences, food habits, and ethnic values. Q**Pcc**

Clear liquid diet

- Consists of foods or fluids that have no residue and are liquid at room temperature.
- Primarily to prevent dehydration and relieve thirst, the diet consists of water and carbohydrates. This diet requires minimal digestion, leaves minimal residue, and is non-gas-forming. It is nutritionally inadequate and should not be used long-term.
- Indications include acute illness, reduction of colon fecal material prior to certain diagnostic tests and procedures, acute gastrointestinal disorders, and some postoperative recovery.
- Acceptable foods are water, tea, coffee, fat-free broth, carbonated beverages, clear juices, ginger ale, and gelatin.

Full liquid diet

- Consists of foods that are liquid at room temperature including plain ice cream and strained cereals. Some facilities include pureed vegetables.
- Offers more variety and nutritional support than a clear liquid diet but might require supplementation of protein and calories if used more than 3 days.
- Indications include a transition from liquid to soft diets, postoperative recovery, acute gastritis, febrile conditions, and intolerance of solid foods.
- Use cautiously with clients who have dysphagia (difficulty swallowing) unless liquids are thickened appropriately. Q**s**
- Many dietary manuals have removed the full liquid diet, so it might be used infrequently.

Blenderized liquid (pureed) diet

- Consists of liquids and foods that are pureed to liquid form.
- The composition and consistency of a pureed diet varies, depending on the client's needs.
- Modify with regard to calories, protein, fat, or other nutrients based on the dietary needs of the client. Q**Pcc**
- Adding broth, milk, gravy, cream, soup, tomato sauce, or fruit juice to foods in place of water provides additional calories and nutritional value.
- Each food is pureed separately to preserve individual flavor.
- Indications include clients who have chewing or swallowing difficulties, oral or facial surgery, and wired jaws.

Soft (bland, low-fiber) diet

- Contains whole foods that are low in fiber, lightly seasoned, and easily digested.
- Food supplements or snacks in between meals add calories.
- Food selections vary and can include smooth, creamy, or crisp textures. Raw fruits and vegetables, coarse breads and cereals, beans, and other potentially gas-forming foods are excluded.
- Indications include clients transitioning between full liquid and regular diets, and those who have acute infections, chewing difficulties, or gastrointestinal disorders.
- Predisposes clients to constipation.

Mechanical soft diet

- A regular diet that is modified in texture. The diet composition is altered for specific nutrient needs.
- Includes foods that require minimal chewing before swallowing (ground meats, canned fruits, softly cooked vegetables).
- Butter, gravies, sugar, or honey can be added to increase calorie intake.
- Excludes harder foods (dried fruits, most raw fruits and vegetables, foods containing seeds and nuts).
- Indications include limited chewing ability; dysphagia, poorly fitting dentures, and clients who are edentulous (without teeth); surgery to the head, neck, or mouth; and strictures of the intestinal tract.

Dysphagia diet

- Prescribed when swallowing is impaired (following a stroke).
- Manifestations of dysphagia are drooling, pocketing food, choking, or gagging.

LEVELS OF SOLID TEXTURES

- **Level 1: Pureed.** Foods are totally pureed to a smooth consistency with a pudding-like texture (pureed fruits, vegetables, meats, soups, scrambled eggs, pudding, custard, applesauce).
- **Level 2: Mechanically altered.** Soft-textured, moist, semi-solid foods that are easily chewed and swallowed (ground meat served with gravy, chicken or tuna salad, well-moistened pancakes with syrup, poached eggs, soft canned or cooked fruit).
- **Level 3: Advanced.** Near-normal textured foods that are moist (moist tender meats or casseroles, breads that are not crusty, moist potatoes, soups, rice, and stuffing). Hard, sticky foods are eliminated.

LEVELS OF LIQUID CONSISTENCIES

- **Thin:** Non-restrictive. Consists of all unthickened beverages and supplements (clear juices, frozen yogurt, ice cream, milk, soda, and broth).
- **Nectar-like:** Liquids that are thin enough to sip through a straw but thicker than water. Consistency of a heavy syrup (nectars, cream soups, buttermilk, and thin milkshakes).
- **Honey-like:** Liquids that do not maintain their shape when poured but are thickened. They can be eaten with a spoon but cannot be sipped through a straw (honey, tomato sauce, and yogurt).
- **Spoon-thick:** Liquids thickened to maintain their shape and need to be eaten with a spoon (pudding, custard, hot cereals).

NURSING ASSESSMENT/DATA COLLECTION AND INTERVENTIONS

- Ongoing assessment parameters include daily weights, prescribed laboratory tests, and an evaluation of a client's nutritional and energy needs and response to diet therapy.
- Observe and document nutritional intake. Perform a calorie count if needed to determine caloric intake and to evaluate adequacy.
- Provide education and support for diet therapy.
- A prescription for a diet as tolerated permits a client's preferences while taking into consideration the client's ability to eat. Assess the client for hunger, appetite, and nausea when planning the most appropriate diet, and consult with a dietitian.
- Dietary intake is progressively increased (from nothing by mouth to clear liquids to regular diet) following a major surgery. Nurses should assess for the return of bowel function (as evidenced by auscultation of bowel sounds and the passage of flatus) before advancing a client's diet. Q_{EBP}

Application Exercises

1. A nurse is caring for a client following an appendectomy who has a postoperative prescription that reads "discontinue NPO status; advance diet as tolerated." Which of the following are appropriate for the nurse to offer the client initially? (Select all that apply.)

   A. Applesauce

   B. Chicken broth

   C. Sherbet

   D. Wheat toast

   E. Cranberry juice

2. A nurse is caring for a client who is to receive a Level 2 dysphagia diet due to a recent stroke. Which of the following dietary selections is most appropriate?

   A. Turkey sandwich

   B. Poached eggs

   C. Peanut butter crackers

   D. Granola

3. A nurse is performing dietary needs assessments for a group of clients. A blenderized liquid diet is appropriate for which of the following clients? (Select all that apply.)

   A. A client who has a wired jaw due to a motor vehicle crash

   B. A client who is 24 hr postoperative following temporomandibular joint repair

   C. A client who has difficulty chewing due to oral surgery

   D. A client who has hypercholesterolemia due to coronary artery disease

   E. A client who is scheduled for a colonoscopy the next morning

4. A nurse is caring for a client who has multiple sclerosis and requires liquids with honey-like thickness. Which of the following foods can the client consume without adding a thickening agent?

   A. Ice cream

   B. Yogurt

   C. Buttermilk

   D. Cream of chicken soup

5. A nurse is assisting a client who has a prescription for a mechanical soft diet with food selections. Which of the following are appropriate selections by the client? (Select all that apply.)

   A. Dried prunes

   B. Ground turkey

   C. Mashed carrots

   D. Fresh strawberries

   E. Cottage cheese

Active Learning Scenario

A nurse is planning care for a newly admitted client who has a prescription for a regular diet. Use the ATI Active Learning Template: Basic Concept to complete this item to include the following sections:

UNDERLYING PRINCIPLES: Identify the indication for a regular diet.

NURSING INTERVENTIONS

- Identify at least two assessments that are appropriate to determine the need for dietary modifications to the regular diet.

- Identify at least two nursing actions that are appropriate to monitor the client's response to diet therapy.

Application Exercises Key

1. A. Applesauce is appropriate once the client's diet begins to advance. It is not appropriate as an initial postoperative selection.
   B. **CORRECT:** Chicken broth is a clear liquid, which is appropriate as an initial selection for a client who is postoperative.
   C. Sherbet is appropriate once the client's diet begins to advance. It is not appropriate as an initial postoperative selection.
   D. Wheat toast is appropriate once the client's diet begins to advance. It is not appropriate as an initial postoperative selection.
   E. **CORRECT:** Cranberry juice is a clear liquid, which is appropriate as an initial selection for a client who is postoperative.

   Ⓝ *NCLEX® Connection: Basic Care and Comfort, Nutrition and Oral Hydration*

2. A. A Level 2 diet requires foods that are moist and semi-solid. A turkey sandwich would be too dry, and breads are not allowed on the Level 2 diet. This would be an appropriate choice for a client receiving a regular diet.
   B. **CORRECT:** A Level 2 diet requires foods that are moist and semi-solid, such as a poached egg.
   C. A Level 2 diet requires foods that are moist and semi-solid. Peanut butter crackers are too sticky and dry for a Level 2 diet. This would be an appropriate choice for a client who is receiving a regular diet.
   D. A Level 2 diet requires foods that are moist and semi-solid. Granola is too hard and crunchy for a client receiving a Level 2 diet.

   Ⓝ *NCLEX® Connection: Reduction of Risk Potential, Potential for Complications of Diagnostic Tests/Treatments/Procedures*

3. A. **CORRECT:** A blenderized liquid diet is appropriate for a client who has a wired jaw.
   B. **CORRECT:** A blenderized liquid diet is appropriate for a client following oral surgery.
   C. **CORRECT:** A blenderized liquid diet is appropriate for a client who has difficulty chewing.
   D. The client's history does not indicate a need for a blenderized liquid diet.
   E. A client who is scheduled for a colonoscopy should receive a clear liquid, rather than a blenderized liquid, diet.

   Ⓝ *NCLEX® Connection: Reduction of Risk Potential, Potential for Alterations in Body Systems*

4. A. Identify ice cream as a thin liquid that can place the client at risk for aspiration.
   B. **CORRECT:** Identify yogurt as a honey-like liquid, because it can be eaten with a spoon but not sipped with a straw. This client can also safely receive spoon-thick liquids.
   C. Identify buttermilk as a nectar-like liquid that can place the client at risk for aspiration.
   D. Identify cream of chicken soup as a nectar-like liquid that can place the client at risk for aspiration.

   Ⓝ *NCLEX® Connection: Basic Care and Comfort, Nutrition and Oral Hydration*

5. A. Dried fruits are excluded from a mechanical soft diet due to potential chewing difficulty.
   B. **CORRECT:** Ground meats require minimal chewing before swallowing and are therefore appropriate for a mechanical soft diet.
   C. **CORRECT:** Mashed carrots require minimal chewing before swallowing and are therefore appropriate for a mechanical soft diet.
   D. Fresh strawberries are excluded from a mechanical soft diet due to seeds and potential chewing difficulty.
   E. **CORRECT:** Cottage cheese requires minimal chewing before swallowing and is therefore appropriate for a mechanical soft diet.

   Ⓝ *NCLEX® Connection: Basic Care and Comfort, Nutrition and Oral Hydration*

Active Learning Scenario Key

Using the ATI Active Learning Template: Basic Concept

UNDERLYING PRINCIPLES: A regular diet is indicated for clients who do not need dietary restrictions.

NURSING INTERVENTIONS

Assessments to determine the need for dietary modification
- Individual preferences
- Food habits
- Ethnic values or practices

Assessments to monitor the client's response to diet therapy
- Obtain daily weight
- Monitor laboratory values
- Monitor energy level
- Observe and document nutritional intake
- Evaluate understanding of diet therapy

Ⓝ *NCLEX® Connection: Physiological Adaptation, Illness Management*

CHAPTER 9

Enteral nutrition (EN) is used when a client cannot consume adequate nutrients and calories orally, but has a gastrointestinal (GI) system that functions at least partially. EN is contraindicated when the GI tract is nonfunctional (paralytic ileus or intestinal obstruction).

EN is administered when a client has a condition (burns, trauma, prolonged intubation, eating disorders, radiation therapy, chemotherapy, liver or renal dysfunction, infection, inflammatory bowel disease) that hinders nutritional status. EN is also administered when a client is neuromuscularly impaired and cannot chew or swallow food.

EN feeding or gavage feeding for an infant is used when an infant is too weak for sucking, unable to coordinate swallowing, and lacks a gag reflex. Gavage feeding is implemented to conserve energy when an infant is attempting to breast feed or bottle feed, but becomes fatigued, weak, or cyanotic.

EN consists of a commercial formula administered by a tube into the stomach or small intestine. Enteral feedings most closely utilize the body's own digestive and metabolic routes. EN can augment an oral diet or be the sole source of nutrition.

ENTERAL FEEDING ROUTES

A client's medical status and the anticipated length of time that a tube feeding will be required determine the type of tube used.

Nasoenteric tubes

Nasoenteric tubes are short-term (less than 3 to 4 weeks).
- **Nasogastric** (NG) tubes are passed through the nose to the stomach.
- **Nasoduodenal** tubes pass from the nose through the stomach and end in the duodenum.
- **Nasojejunal** tubes pass from the nose through the stomach and end in the jejunum.
- Nasoduodenal and nasojejunal tubes are used in clients who are at risk for aspiration or who have delayed gastric emptying (gastroparesis).
- For an infant, a feeding tube is inserted from the nares or mouth into the stomach. This flexible tube can remain taped in place for up to 30 days.

Ostomies

Ostomies are placed for clients requiring long-term enteral feeding, who are at high risk for aspiration or when a nasal obstruction makes insertion through the nose impossible. An ostomy is a surgically created opening (stoma); ostomies can be used to deliver feedings directly into the stomach or intestines.

Gastrostomy tubes are endoscopically or surgically inserted into the stomach.
- A percutaneous endoscopic gastrostomy (PEG) tube is placed with the aid of an endoscope.
- An alternative to the PEG tube is a skin-level gastrostomy tube, which is known as a low-profile gastrostomy device. It is more comfortable, longer-lasting, and fully immersible in water. Checking for residual is more difficult with this device because of the close proximity of the button on the skin.
- Gastrostomy tube feedings are generally well-tolerated because the stomach chamber holds and releases feedings in a physiologic manner that promotes effective digestion. As a result, dumping syndrome is usually avoided.

Jejunostomy tubes are surgically inserted into the jejunal portion of the small intestine (jejunum).

ENTERAL FEEDING FORMULAS

- Commercial products are preferred over home-blended ingredients because the nutrient composition, consistency and safety can be better insured.
- Standard and elemental formulas are the two primary types of enteral feeding formulas available. They are categorized by the complexity of the proteins included.
- Other formula types include disease-specific (COPD, kidney disease, immunocompromise) and modular formulas that typically contain a single nutrient (protein, carbohydrates, fat).

Standard formulas

- Also called polymeric or intact, these formulas are composed of whole proteins (milk, meat, eggs) or protein isolates.
- They require a functioning gastrointestinal tract.
- Most provide 1 to 2 cal/mL.

Elemental formulas

- These formulas are made up of nutrients that are partially or fully hydrolyzed or broken down.
- These formulas are used for clients who have a partially functioning gastrointestinal tract, or those who have an impaired ability to digest and absorb foods (inflammatory bowel disease, liver failure, cystic fibrosis, pancreatic disorders, and short-gut syndrome).
- Most provide 1.0 to 1.5 cal/mL. High-calorie formulas provide 1.5 to 2.0 cal/mL. Partially hydrolyzed formulas provide other nutrients in simpler forms that require little or no digestion.

PACKAGING

Tube feedings can be packaged in cans or prefilled bags.
- Prefilled bags and administration tubing should be discarded every 24 hr or according to facility policy, even if they are not empty.
- Cans can be used to add formula to a generic bag to infuse via a pump, or for feedings directly from a syringe.

DETERMINING APPROPRIATE FORMULA

Caloric density determines the volume of the formula necessary to meet the caloric needs of a client (1.0 to 1.2 cal/mL).

Water content in formulas with 1.0 cal/mL should be 850 mL water per 1 L formula. Higher-calorie formulas have lower water content. The client might need additional free water to meet hydration needs.

Osmolality of the formula is determined by the amount of dissolved particles of sugars, amino acids, and electrolytes.
- Osmolality is increased if the formula contains more digested protein.
- Hydrolyzed or partially hydrolyzed (predigested) formulas are higher in osmolality than standard formulas. They are also lactose-free.

Fiber and residue content
- Standard formulas are low in residue which makes them less likely to produce abdominal distention or gas. These products are optimal for clients who have been on bowel rest, are postoperative following bowel surgery, or have GI related disease processes. Hydrolyzed formulas are considered residue-free.
- Standard formulas that are enriched with fiber are recommended for clients who have constipation or diarrhea to normalize bowel movements.

The presence of **other nutrients** include fats and carbohydrates, which can be modified according to a client's disease processes (respiratory disease, malabsorption, diabetes mellitus, kidney disease).

ENTERAL FEEDING DELIVERY METHODS

The delivery method is dependent on the type and location of the feeding tube, type of formula administered, and the client's medical status and GI function.

Continuous infusion method

Formula is administered at a continuous rate over a 24-hr period.
- Infusion pumps help ensure consistent flow rates.
- This method is recommended for critically ill clients because of its association with smaller residual volumes, and a lower risk of aspiration and diarrhea.
- Many facilities require measuring gastric residual volume (GRV) every 4 to 6 hr. Other facilities are moving away from this practice, as there is insufficient evidence to support it.
- Feeding tubes should be flushed with at least 30 mL of water every 4 hr to maintain tube patency and provide hydration.
- Check facility policy regarding withholding feedings for high gastric residual volume (GRV). Typically, the amount is more than 250 mL on two consecutive measurements for an adult or more than one-fourth the prescribed volume for children.

Cyclic feeding

- Formula is administered at a continuous rate for 8 to 20 hr, often during sleeping hours.
- Often used for transition from total EN to oral intake.

Intermittent tube feeding

Formula is administered every 4 to 6 hr in equal portions of 250 to 400 mL, typically over a 30- to 60-min time frame, usually by gravity drip or an electronic pump. Feeding times can range from 20 to 90 min.
- This is often used for noncritical clients, home tube feedings, and clients in rehabilitation.
- Feeding resembles normal pattern of nutrient intake.
- Facilities might require measurement prior to initiating the feeding and held if the amount is greater than the amount stated in facility policy or prescription.

Bolus feeding

A variation of intermittent feeding using a large syringe attached to the feeding tube. The rate of administration and volume varies depending upon the client's needs and tolerance. Volumes ranging from 250 to 400 mL can be administered over a period of at least 15 min four to six times daily. Facility policies may provide further guidance regarding administration rates.
- The rate of administration for a premature or small infant should be no greater than 5 mL every 10 min, and 10 mL/min in older infants and children.
- Bolus feedings are delivered directly into the stomach; they are contraindicated for tubes placed into the jejunum or duodenum. They can be poorly tolerated and can cause dumping syndrome.

NURSING ACTIONS

PREPARATION OF THE CLIENT

- Prior to instilling enteral feeding, tube placement should be verified by radiography. The tube should then be marked with indelible ink or adhesive tape where it exits the nose and documented.
- Measure the tube each shift and prior to each feeding to ensure the tube has not migrated. Aspirating gastric contents and measuring pH levels are not considered reliable methods of verifying initial placement. Q_EBP
- Verify the presence of bowel sounds.
- To maintain feeding tube patency, it is flushed routinely with warm water.
- Check gastric residuals if required by the facility, typically every 4 to 6 hr. In some cases, policy or prescription will indicate whether to return the contents to the client's stomach or to hold or reduce feedings.
  - The volume that indicates a need for intervention for adults ranges from 100 to 500 mL in a single measurement, or at least 250 mL on two consecutive checks.
  - Returning residual contents to the stomach prevents electrolyte and fluid imbalance. However, returning large volumes could increase the risk for complications.
- The head of the bed should be elevated at least 30° during feedings and for at least 30 to 60 min afterward to lessen the risk of aspiration. Q_s
- Burp the infant following the feeding if the infant's condition allows.
- Begin with a small volume of full-strength formula. Increase volume in intervals as tolerated until the desired volume is achieved.
- Administer the feeding solution at room temperature to decrease gastrointestinal discomfort.
- Do not heat formulas in a microwave as this can result in uneven temperatures within the solution.

BASELINE PARAMETERS

- Obtain height, weight, and body mass index.
- Monitor blood urea nitrogen (BUN), albumin, hemoglobin, hematocrit, glucose, and electrolyte levels.
- A registered dietitian will work with the provider to evaluate nutritional and energy needs.
- Verify gastrointestinal function. Dysfunction of the GI tract can indicate a need for alternate forms of nutrition.

ONGOING CARE

- Monitor daily weights and I&O.
- Obtain gastric residuals every 4 to 6 hr.
- Monitor electrolytes, BUN, creatinine, minerals, and CBC.
- Monitor the tube site for manifestations of infection or intolerance (pain, redness, swelling, drainage).
- Monitor the character and frequency of bowel movements.
- When appropriate, administer medications through a feeding tube.
  - Feeding should be stopped prior to administering medications.
  - The tubing should be flushed with water (15 to 30 mL) before and after the medication is administered, and between each medication if more than one is administered.
  - Medications should only be dissolved in water.
  - Liquid medications should be used when possible.
    - For an infant or child, the volume of water to flush is 1.5 times the amount predetermined to flush an unused feeding tube of the same size.
    - More water can be required to flush the tubing following some medications (suspensions).

INTERVENTIONS

- Weaning occurs as oral consumption increases. Enteral feedings can be discontinued when the client consumes two-thirds of protein and calorie needs orally for 3 to 5 days.
- A client who is NPO will require meticulous oral care.
- A client can require nutritional support service at home for long-term EN. A interprofessional team comprised of a nurse, dietitian, pharmacist, and the provider monitors the client's weight, electrolyte balance, and overall physical condition. Q_TC
- Transitioning from EN to an oral diet requires the client to receive adequate nutrition as food items are reintroduced.
  - Begin the transition process by stopping the EN for 1 hr before a meal.
  - Slowly increase the frequency of the meals until the client is eating up to six small meals daily.
  - When oral intake equals 500 to 750 cal/day, the continuous tube feeding is administered only during the night.

COMPLICATIONS

Gastrointestinal complications

- Constipation, diarrhea, cramping, pain, abdominal distention, dumping syndrome, nausea, and vomiting.
- Dumping syndrome occurs due to rapid emptying of the formula into the small intestine, resulting in a fluid shift. Manifestations include dizziness, rapid pulse, diaphoresis, pallor, and lightheadedness.

NURSING ACTIONS
- Consider a change in formula.
- Decrease the flow rate or total volume of the infusion.
- Increase the volume of free water if constipated.
- Administer the EN at room temperature.
- Take measures to prevent bacterial contamination.

Mechanical complications

Tube misplacement or dislodgement; aspiration; irritation and leakage at the insertion site; irritation of the nose, esophagus, and mucosa; and clogging of the feeding tube.

NURSING ACTIONS
- Confirm tube placement prior to feedings.
- Elevate the head of the bed at least 30° during feedings and maintain the client in this position for approximately 60 min following completion of the feeding.
- Administer bolus feedings over a period of at least 15 min and according to client tolerance.
- Flush the tubing with at least 30 mL of water every 4 hr for continuous infusion, after measuring gastric residual, before and after bolus feedings, and between each medication administration.
- Unclog tubing using gentle pressure with 30 to 50 mL warm water in a 60 mL piston syringe. Carbonated beverages are not approved for fixing a clogged tube. Commercially-made products are available and have been shown to effectively dissolve clotted formula.
- Do not mix medications with the formula.

Metabolic complications

Include dehydration, hyperglycemia, electrolyte imbalances, fluid overload, refeeding syndrome, rapid weight gain

NURSING ACTIONS
- Provide adequate amounts of free water.
- Consider changing formula to one that is isotonic.
- Restrict fluids if fluid overload occurs.
- Monitor electrolytes, blood glucose, and weights.
- Monitor respiratory, cardiovascular, and neurologic status.
- Administer insulin per prescribed protocol for hyperglycemia.

Refeeding syndrome

A potentially fatal complication that occurs when a client who is in a starvation state is started on enteral nutrition. The risk is greater with parenteral nutrition than enteral.

Food poisoning

Can result due to bacterial contamination of formula

NURSING ACTIONS: **Prevent bacterial contamination.**
- Wash hands before handling formula or enteral products.
- Clean equipment and tops of formula cans.
- Use closed feeding systems.
- Cover and label unused cans with the client's name, room number, date, and time of opening.
- Refrigerate unused portions promptly for up to 24 hr.
- Replace the feeding bag, administration tubing, and any equipment used to mix the formula every 24 hr.
- Fill generic bags with only 4 hr worth of formula.

Application Exercises

1. A nurse is discussing the use of a low-profile gastrostomy device with the guardian of a child who is receiving an enteral feeding. Which of the following is an appropriate statement by the nurse?
   A. "The device is usually comfortable for children."
   B. "Checking residual is much easier with this device."
   C. "This access requires less maintenance than a traditional nasal tube."
   D. "Mobility of the child is limited with this device."

2. A nurse is teaching a client who is starting continuous feedings about the various types of enteral nutrition (EN) formulas. Which of the following should the nurse include in the teaching?
   A. Formula rich in fiber is recommended when starting EN.
   B. Standard formula contains whole protein.
   C. Hydrolyzed formula is recommended for a full-functioning GI tract.
   D. The high-calorie formula has increased water content.

3. A nurse is instructing a client on how to administer cyclic enteral feedings at home. Which of the following information should the nurse include?
   A. "Give a feeding every 6 hours."
   B. "Set the feeding up before you go to bed."
   C. "Weigh yourself daily."
   D. "Flush the tube with a carbonated beverage to dislodge clogs."
   E. "Ensure your head is elevated to 15 degrees during administration."

4. A nurse is administering bolus enteral feedings to a client who has malnutrition. Which of the following are appropriate nursing interventions? (Select all that apply.)
   A. Verify the presence of bowel sounds.
   B. Flush the feeding tube with warm water.
   C. Elevate the head of the bed 20°.
   D. Administer the feeding at room temperature.
   E. Instill the formula over 60 min.

5. A nurse is preparing to administer intermittent enteral feeding to a client. Which of the following are appropriate nursing interventions? (Select all that apply.)
   A. Fill the feeding bag with 24 hr worth of formula.
   B. Discard feeding equipment after 24 hr.
   C. Place any unused formula in open cans in the refrigerator.
   D. Flush the feeding tube every 4 hr.
   E. Elevate the head of the client's bed for 15 min after administration.

Active Learning Scenario

A nurse is providing information to a client on complications that can occur when administering an enteral nutrition. What information should the nurse include in the teaching? Use the ATI Active Learning Template: Basic Concept to complete this item to include the following.

RELATED CONTENT: Identify three complications. List two nursing interventions for each complication.

Application Exercises Key

1. A. **CORRECT:** The gastrostomy device is more comfortable for children because of the close proximity of the button on the skin.
   B. Checking for residual is more difficult with this device because of the close proximity of the button on the skin.
   C. Instruct the guardian to provide regular stoma care, and give information about flushing the tube.
   D. The mobility of the child is increased because of the close proximity of the button on the skin.

   Ⓝ *NCLEX® Connection: Basic Care and Comfort, Nutrition and Oral Hydration*

2. A. Residual-free formula without fiber is recommended when starting EN to minimize abdominal distention from increased flatus.
   B. **CORRECT:** A standard formula contains whole protein (milk, meat, eggs) and requires a full-functioning GI tract.
   C. Hydrolyzed formula is recommended for a partially functioning digestive tract or for those who have impaired ability to digest and absorb foods.
   D. Formula high in calories is low in water content.

   Ⓝ *NCLEX® Connection: Basic Care and Comfort, Nutrition and Oral Hydration*

3. A. Include this instruction for a client who is prescribed intermittent feedings.
   B. **CORRECT:** Many clients administer cyclic feedings during sleeping hours, so they are free during the daytime to do other things.
   C. **CORRECT:** The client should obtain a daily weight while receiving enteral nutrition.
   D. Have the client notify the provider if the tube is clogged to obtain a commercial remedy to dislodge the tube.
   E. Tell the client to elevate the head 30° or more during administration.

   Ⓝ *NCLEX® Connection: Basic Care and Comfort, Nutrition and Oral Hydration*

4. A. **CORRECT:** Verify the presence of bowel sounds prior to a bolus feeding to ensure the bowel is functioning.
   B. **CORRECT:** Flush the feeding tube to ensure patency before administering a bolus feeding.
   C. Elevate the client's head of bed at least 30° prior to a bolus feeding to decrease the risk of aspiration.
   D. **CORRECT:** Administer the bolus feeding at room temperature to prevent abdominal cramping.
   E. Instill the formula in a shorter time period, at least 15 min.

   Ⓝ *NCLEX® Connection: Basic Care and Comfort, Nutrition and Oral Hydration*

5. A. The feeding bag should be filled with only enough formula for 4 hr to prevent bacterial contamination.
   B. **CORRECT:** Feeding equipment, such as the bag holding the formula and the tubing, should be discarded every 24 hr to prevent bacterial contamination.
   C. **CORRECT:** The unused portion of formula should be refrigerated up to 24 hr to prevent bacterial contamination.
   D. **CORRECT:** Flushing the feeding tube every 4 hr maintains patency.
   E. Elevate the head of the client's bed for 30 to 60 min following administration to prevent aspiration.

   Ⓝ *NCLEX® Connection: Basic Care and Comfort, Nutrition and Oral Hydration*

Active Learning Scenario Key

Using the ATI Active Learning Template: Basic Concept
RELATED CONTENT

Gastrointestinal disturbance
- Increase the amount of free fluid if constipated.
- Consider a change to formula with enriched fiber if constipated.
- Decrease the flow rate if cramping occurs.
- Give the formula at room temperature.

Feeding tube obstruction
- Flush the tubing with at least 30 mL of water every 4 hr.
- Flush before and after feedings and medication.
- Use a piston syringe with 50 mL of warm water to unclog the tubing.
- Carbonated beverages are not approved to clear clogged enteral tubes.

Food poisoning
- Wash hands before handling the formula or equipment.
- Clean tops of formula containers.
- Cover and refrigerate formula up to 24 hr.
- Replace the feeding bag and administration tubing every 24 hr.

Ⓝ *NCLEX® Connection: Reduction of Risk Potential, Potential for Complications of Diagnostic Tests/Treatments/Procedures*

CHAPTER 10

Total Parenteral Nutrition

Parenteral nutrition (PN) is used when a client's gastrointestinal tract is not functioning, or when a client cannot physically or psychologically consume sufficient nutrients orally or enterally. Based upon the client's nutritional needs and anticipated duration of therapy, PN can be given as either total parenteral nutrition (TPN) or peripheral parenteral nutrition (PPN).

TPN provides a nutritionally complete solution. It can be used when caloric needs are very high, when long-term therapy is indicated, or when the solution to be administered is hypertonic (composed of greater than 10% dextrose). It can only be administered in a central vein.

PPN is administered for up to 14 days into a peripheral vein. It is nutritionally incomplete because it has a low dextrose content. It is indicated for clients who require short-term nutritional support with fewer calories per day. The solution must be isotonic and contain no more than 10% dextrose and 5% amino acids.

COMPONENTS OF PARENTERAL NUTRITION SOLUTIONS

PN includes amino acids, dextrose, electrolytes, vitamins, and trace elements in sterile water. Fats (lipids) are added to the parenteral solution or given as an intermittent infusion.

Carbohydrate or dextrose solutions are available in concentrations of 2.5% to 10% for PPN and up to 70% for TPN.
- A higher concentration of dextrose is often prescribed for a client on fluid restrictions.
- A lower-dextrose concentration can be used to help control hyperglycemia.

Electrolytes, vitamins, and trace elements are essential for normal body functions. The amounts added are dependent upon the client's blood chemistry values and physical findings, which are used to determine the quantity of electrolytes. Additional vitamin K can be added to the PN solution.

Lipids (fats) are available in concentrations of 10%, 20%, and 30%. Lipids are formulated from a combination of soybean oil and/or safflower oil, and egg phospholipids, which gives lipids a milky or opaque appearance.
- IV lipids are contraindicated for clients who have severe hyperlipidemia, severe hepatic disease, or an allergy to soybean oil, eggs, or safflower oil.
- Lipid emulsion provides the needed calories when dextrose concentration must be reduced due to fluid restrictions or persistent hyperglycemia. They also correct or prevent essential fatty acid deficiency.
- Lipid emulsion provides the calories without increasing the osmolality of the PN solution.
- Total nutrient admixtures are available that combine lipids into the PN solution containing dextrose and amino acids, rather than administering the solutions separately. Not all facilities use this three-in-one solution.
  ○ Three-in-one infusions reduce body carbon dioxide production and buildup of fat in the liver.

Protein is provided as a mixture of essential and nonessential amino acids and is available in concentrations of 3% to 20%. The client's estimated requirements and liver and kidney function determine the amount of protein provided.

Other substances can be added to the PN solution by pharmacy services.
- Insulin can be added to reduce the potential for hyperglycemia.
- Heparin can be added to prevent fibrin buildup on the catheter tip.
- Glutamine, antioxidants, prebiotics, or probiotics might be prescribed based on individual client needs.

   ! Administering any IV medication through a PN IV line or port is contraindicated.

INDICATIONS

DIAGNOSES
- TPN is commonly used in clients who need intense nutritional support for an extended period of time, including clients undergoing treatment for cancer, bowel disorders, those who are critically ill, and those suffering from trauma or extensive burns, as these conditions are associated with high caloric requirements.
- PPN can be used when the client is unable to consume enough calories to meet metabolic needs or when nutritional support is needed for a short time.
- Clients can receive PN at home as nutrition replacement or to supplement nutrition. Typically, the client will have a tunneled catheter, and feedings can occur while the client sleeps.

DESIRED THERAPEUTIC OUTCOMES
- Improved nutritional status
- Weight maintenance or gain
- Positive nitrogen balance

EVIDENCE SUPPORTING EFFECTIVENESS

- Daily weight: Maintenance of baseline or gain of up to 1 kg/day
- Increases in prealbumin level (expected reference range of 15 to 36 mg/dL)
- Blood urea nitrogen level within the expected reference range (10 to 20 mg/dL)

CONSIDERATIONS

PREPARATION OF THE CLIENT

- Prior to initiating PN, review the client's weight, BMI, nutritional status, diagnosis, and current laboratory data. This can include CBC, blood chemistry profile, PT/aPTT, iron, total iron-binding capacity, lipid profile, liver function tests, electrolyte panel, BUN, prealbumin and albumin level, creatinine, blood glucose, and platelet count.
- Assess the client's educational needs.
- Use an electronic infusion device to prevent the accidental overload of a solution.
- A micron filter on the IV tubing is required when administering PN solution. This filter is not added to the IV tubing when administering a lipid emulsion.
- Evaluate for allergies to soybeans, safflower, or eggs if lipids are prescribed.

ONGOING CARE

Nursing care is focused on preventing complications through consistent monitoring. Specific monitoring guidelines vary among health care facilities.

- Parameters can include I&O, daily weights, vital signs, pertinent laboratory values (e.g., electrolytes), and evaluation of the client's underlying condition. This data is used to determine the client's response to therapy, whether the formulation of the solution is correct, and to prevent nutrient deficiencies or toxicities.
- Monitor blood and urine glucose as prescribed and per facility guidelines. Sliding scale insulin can treat or prevent hyperglycemia, or regular insulin can be added to the PN solution.
- Monitor flow rate carefully.
  - Administering the solution too slowly will fail to meet the client's nutritional needs.
  - Administering the infusion too rapidly can cause hyperosmolar diuresis, which can lead to dehydration, hypovolemic shock, seizures, coma, and death.
  - To avoid hypoglycemia, an IV of dextrose 10% to 20% in water is administered if the PN solution is unavailable.
  - Do not attempt to increase the rate of the PN solution to "catch up." Hyperglycemia, hyperosmolar diuresis, and fluid overload can occur if the PN solution is increased when available.

- Monitor for "cracking" of TPN solution. This occurs if the calcium or phosphorous content is high or if poor-salt albumin is added. A "cracked" TPN solution has an oily appearance or a layer of fat on top of the solution and should not be used. Qs
- Verify the prescription of the PN solution with a second nurse prior to administration.
- If the PN solution is prepared and stored in the refrigerator, allow it to come to room temperature for 1 hr prior to administering it.
- Maintain strict aseptic techniques to reduce the risk of infection. The high dextrose content of PN contributes to bacterial growth.
- Use sterile technique when changing central line dressing and tubing. Change the bag and IV tubing for the dextrose solution every 24 hr unless facility policy differs. With intermittent IV lipid infusions, ensure the solution does not hang more than 12 hr to prevent microbial growth.
- Ensure lipid infusion is stopped 12 hr prior to obtaining a blood specimen for triglycerides to ensure accurate results.

NURSING ACTIONS

- Ask the provider about giving some enteral substance during long-term PN administration, such as diluted juice, to prevent atrophy of the gastrointestinal tract. QEBP
- PN should be discontinued as soon as possible to avoid potential complications, but not until the client's enteral or oral intake can provide 60% or more of estimated caloric requirements.

  ! Discontinuation should be done gradually to avoid rebound hypoglycemia.

- During transition, the client will need enteral or oral nutrition. Oral nutrition usually begins with clear liquids that are low in fat or substances that might irritate the client's gastrointestinal tract. The client might not have an appetite for 1 to 2 weeks, so PN infusion will need to continue until the client can take in adequate calories through other means.
- Educate the client and family regarding home PN, including aseptic preparation and administration techniques, blood glucose monitoring, and criteria to evaluate for complications.

COMPLICATIONS

Infection and sepsis are evidenced by a fever or elevated WBC count. Infection can result from contamination of the catheter during insertion, contaminated solution, or a long-term indwelling catheter.

Metabolic complications include hyperglycemia, hypoglycemia, hyperkalemia, hypophosphatemia, hypocalcemia, dehydration (related to hyperosmolar diuresis resulting from hyperglycemia), and fluid overload (as evidenced by weight gain greater than 1 kg/day and edema).

Mechanical complications include catheter misplacement resulting in pneumothorax or hemothorax (evidenced by shortness of breath, diminished or absent breath sounds), arterial puncture, catheter embolus, air embolus, thrombosis, obstruction, and bolus infusion due to incorrectly set or malfunctioning electronic pumps.

Refeeding syndrome occurs when the body rapidly changes from catabolic (seen in starvation states) to anabolic metabolism when nutrition is started. It is characterized by fluid and electrolyte imbalances (potassium, magnesium, phosphate). Manifestations include shallow respirations, confusion, seizures, weakness, cardiac rhythm changes, fluid retention, and acidosis.

NURSING ACTIONS

- Monitor for manifestations of fever, chills, increased WBCs, and redness around the catheter insertion site.
- Use strict aseptic technique when setting up the IV tubing, changing the site dressing, and accessing or deaccessing the IV access. Change the PN bag and tubing set every 24 hr or per facility protocol.
- Monitor blood glucose per prescription or facility policy.
- Administer sliding scale insulin or plan for insulin to be added to the TPN solution to treat hyperglycemia.
- Plan to administer additional dextrose to treat hypoglycemia.
- Monitor daily weights, I&O, and oral intake of nutrients.
- Notify the provider of weight gain greater than 1 kg/day.
- Anticipate a decrease in the concentration of the solution, rate of administration, or volume of lipid emulsion to treat weight gain.

Active Learning Scenario

A nurse is teaching a client about complications that can occur when receiving total parenteral nutrition (TPN). What should the nurse include in the teaching? Use the ATI Active Learning Template: Basic Concept to complete this item to include the following.

RELATED CONTENT: Identify three complications of TPN. Describe two nursing actions related to each complication.

Application Exercises

1. A nurse is planning care for a client who has a new prescription for peripheral parenteral nutrition (PPN). Which of the following actions should the nurse include in the plan of care? (Select all that apply.)
   A. Examine trends in weight loss.
   B. Review prealbumin finding.
   C. Administer an IV solution of 20% dextrose.
   D. Add a micron filter to IV tubing.
   E. Use an IV infusion pump.

2. A charge nurse is providing information about fat emulsion added to total parenteral nutrition (TPN) to a group of nurses. Which of the following statements by the charge nurse are appropriate? (Select all that apply.)
   A. "Concentration of lipid emulsion can be up to 30%."
   B. "Adding lipid emulsion gives the solution a milky appearance."
   C. "Check for allergies to soybean oil."
   D. "Lipid emulsion prevents essential fatty acid deficiency."
   E. "Lipids provide calories by increasing the osmolality of the PN solution."

3. A charge nurse is teaching a group of nurses about medication compatibility with TPN. Which of the following statements should the charge nurse make?
   A. "Use the Y-port on the TPN IV tubing to administer antibiotics."
   B. "Regular insulin can be added to the TPN solution."
   C. "Administer heparin through a port on the TPN tubing."
   D. "Administer vitamin K IV bolus via a Y-port on the TPN tubing."

4. A nurse is preparing to administer lipid emulsion and notes a layer of fat floating in the IV solution bag. Which of the following actions should the nurse take?
   A. Shake the bag to mix the fat.
   B. Turn the bag upside down one time.
   C. Return the bag to the pharmacy.
   D. Administer the bag of solution as it is.

5. A nurse is caring for a client who is receiving TPN through a central venous access device, but the next bag of solution is not available for administration at this time. Which of the following is an appropriate action by the nurse?
   A. Administer 20% dextrose in water IV until the next bag is available.
   B. Slow the infusion rate of the current bag until the solution is available.
   C. Monitor for hyperglycemia.
   D. Monitor for hyperosmolar diuresis.

1. A. **CORRECT:** Examining trends in weight loss will help to evaluate the outcome of PPN.
    B. **CORRECT:** Reviewing the prealbumin finding will determine nutritional deficiency over a short period of time.
    C. An IV solution of 20% dextrose is administered only as TPN using a central vein.
    D. **CORRECT:** A micron filter is always used when infusing PN solution.
    E. **CORRECT:** An IV infusion pump is always used to regulate the flow and provide accurate delivery of the PN solution.

    ⓝ *NCLEX® Connection: Pharmacological and Parenteral Therapies, Total Parenteral Nutrition (TPN)*

2. A. **CORRECT:** Lipid emulsion is available in 10%, 20%, and 30% concentrations depending upon the client's carbohydrate and caloric needs.
    B. **CORRECT:** The lipid emulsion is formulated from safflower and/or soybean oils and egg phospholipid, making the solution appear milky.
    C. **CORRECT:** Lipid emulsion is formulated from safflower and/or soybean oil and egg phospholipid. The nurse should check for allergies to these ingredients.
    D. **CORRECT:** Lipid emulsion is used for additional calories as concentrated energy and to prevent essential fatty acid deficiency.
    E. Lipids provide the calories needed without increasing osmolality of the PN solution.

    ⓝ *NCLEX® Connection: Pharmacological and Parenteral Therapies, Total Parenteral Nutrition (TPN)*

3. A. Administering any IV medication through a Y-port on the TPN line is contraindicated.
    B. **CORRECT:** Regular insulin may be added to the TPN solution to decrease hyperglycemia.
    C. Heparin may be added to the TPN solution to decrease clot formation in the cannula, but it is not injected directly into a port on the TPN tubing.
    D. Vitamin K can be added to the TPN solution, but it should not be administered IV bolus through the TPN IV line.

    ⓝ *NCLEX® Connection: Pharmacological and Parenteral Therapies, Total Parenteral Nutrition (TPN)*

4. A. Shaking the bag is not an appropriate action because "cracking" of the solution has occurred and it should not be administered.
    B. Turning the solution upside down does not resolve the problem because cracking of the TPN has occurred and it should not be administered.
    C. **CORRECT:** Returning the solution to the pharmacy is an appropriate action by the nurse because cracking of the solution has occurred and it should not be administered. The pharmacist and provider will need to adjust the formulation of the solution to prevent cracking.
    D. Administering the solution as it is would not be an appropriate nursing action because cracking of the solution has occurred. Infusion of a cracked solution can lead to fat or particulate embolisms.

    ⓝ *NCLEX® Connection: Pharmacological and Parenteral Therapies, Nutrition and Oral Hydration*

5. A. **CORRECT:** Administering 20% dextrose in water IV until the TPN solution is available will prevent hypoglycemia.
    B. Decreasing the rate of the TPN solution is not an appropriate action because the decreased rate can cause hypoglycemia.
    C. The client should be monitored for hypoglycemia when the TPN solution is not infusing and adequate glucose is not provided.
    D. Monitor the client for hyperosmolar diuresis when the TPN solution has infused too fast.

    ⓝ *NCLEX® Connection: Pharmacological and Parenteral Therapies, Total Parenteral Nutrition (TPN)*

Using the ATI Active Learning Template: Basic Concept
RELATED CONTENT

Infection and sepsis
- Monitor for manifestations of fever, chills, increased WBCs, and redness around catheter insertion site.
- Use aseptic technique when setting up the IV tubing and accessing or deaccessing the port.
- Use sterile technique when changing central line dressing and tubing.
- Change the PN bag and tubing set every 24 hr or per facility protocol.

Hyperglycemia
- Administer sliding scale insulin or plan for insulin to be added to the TPN solution.
- Monitor blood glucose.

Hypoglycemia
- Inform the provider and plan to give additional dextrose.
- Monitor frequent blood glucose.

Weight gain greater than 1 kg/day
- Inform the provider and anticipate a decrease in the concentration, rate of administration or volume of lipid emulsion.
- Monitor the client's intake of oral nutrients.

ⓝ *NCLEX® Connection: Pharmacological and Parenteral Therapies, Nutrition and Oral Hydration*

When reviewing the following chapters, keep in mind the relevant topics and tasks of the NCLEX outline, in particular:

Health Promotion and Maintenance

HEALTH PROMOTION/DISEASE PREVENTION
Identify risk factors for disease/illness.

Educate the client on actions to promote/ maintain health and prevent disease.

HEALTH SCREENING: Perform targeted screening assessments.

HIGH-RISK BEHAVIORS: Assist the client to identify behaviors/risks that may impact health.

Basic Care and Comfort

ELIMINATION: Assess and manage client with an alteration in elimination.

NUTRITION AND ORAL HYDRATION
Provide nutritional supplements as needed.

Evaluate the impact of disease/illness on the nutritional status of a client.

Physiological Adaptation

ALTERATIONS IN BODY SYSTEMS: Implement interventions to address side/adverse effects of radiation therapy.

ILLNESS MANAGEMENT: Educate the client about managing illness.

FLUID AND ELECTROLYTE IMBALANCES: Manage the care of the client with a fluid and electrolyte imbalance.

Reduction of Risk Potential

POTENTIAL FOR ALTERATIONS IN BODY SYSTEMS:
Identify client potential for aspiration.

SYSTEM SPECIFIC ASSESSMENTS: Assess the client for signs of hypoglycemia or hyperglycemia

UNIT 3   ALTERATIONS IN NUTRITION

CHAPTER 11 *Barriers to Adequate Nutrition*

Many individuals have difficulty consuming a nutritional or prescribed diet due to factors that create a barrier. Medical, psychological, and social factors can all create nutritional barriers. Approximately 30% to 50% of clients in acute care facilities are malnourished upon admission or during part of their hospital stay.

It is important for nurses to recognize these factors as nutritional education will be ineffective if a client lacks the necessary resources to follow through on recommendations.

NUTRITIONAL BARRIERS AND NURSING INTERVENTIONS

Poor dentition

Poor dentition (dental caries, poorly fitting dentures) is a potential problem for clients across the lifespan.
- Children who do not have access to dental care or tools (toothbrush, toothpaste) can have caries that impair the ability to chew.
- Adults who have lost teeth or have teeth that need removal or repair have an impaired ability to chew.
- After an adult has teeth removed, it can be difficult to adjust to dentures.

NURSING CARE
- School screenings can help identify children who need dental attention, and can facilitate the referral process.
- Provide children with information about healthy snacks that are low in sugar.
- Advise children and adults to limit consumption of processed carbohydrates, which can stick to teeth and increase the risk for dental caries.
- Encourage children and adults to use a fluoridated tooth paste and have fluoride applied to their teeth. Q_{EBP}
- Perform a basic dental screening for clients admitted to acute or long-term care facilities to identify issues that can affect the ability to properly eat.
- Consult a dietitian or nutritionist to assist with meal and diet planning, as well as for recommendations on nutritional supplements. Q_{TC}

Low socioeconomic status and lack of access

The lack of money to purchase healthy foods or foods required for a specific diet can be a barrier to maintaining a proper diet.
- Nutritious foods (fresh fruit, vegetables) tend to be more expensive than canned and boxed foods.
- Canned, boxed, and processed foods (lunch meats and frozen meals) are usually high in calories and salt, and often contain a higher fat, sodium, and simple carbohydrate content. These are poor choices for clients on calorie- or sodium-restricted diets.
- The lack of money to purchase necessary food can lead to malnutrition or obesity if canned and boxed foods are selected.
- The lack of transportation to grocery stores is a barrier if the client does not have a car or is not licensed to drive.
- Food deserts occur in low-socioeconomic areas where a person lives more than 1 mile from a food source in the urban area, or more than 10 miles in a rural area.

NURSING CARE
- Refer the client to a dietitian who can discuss food options and substitutions that are appropriate.
- Instruct the client that frozen fruits and vegetables can be an affordable option, and are maintained longer in the freezer.
- Educate clients on how to read food labels to be aware of nutritional, caloric, and sodium values of the food they are consuming.
- Contact social services regarding the client's access to food. Investigate the availability of a nutrition program that provides a meal for clients within a community. Q_{TC}

Cognitive disorders

Cognitive disorders (dementia, Alzheimer's disease [AD]) can have a significant impact on nutritional status.
- Clients who have dementia or AD can experience impairments in memory and judgment, making shopping, food selection, and food preparation difficult.
- As dementia and AD progress, clients might refuse to eat or choose a small selection of food that might not provide adequate nutrition.

NURSING CARE
- If the client lives independently, encourage shopping with a friend or family member and following a shopping list.
- Monitor for vitamin and mineral deficits, and evaluate the need for nutritional supplements.
- Contact social services regarding the availability of food or meal delivery to the client's home.
- If the client lives in a care facility, provide a menu with minimal but nutritious options.
- Serve meals at the same time and in the same location surrounded by the same people. Keep environmental distractions to a minimum.
- Provide snacks in between meals if mealtime intake is inadequate.
- Cut food into small pieces if the client has difficulty chewing food. Remind the client to chew and then swallow. Lightly stroking the chin and throat can help promote swallowing. Q_S

Altered sensory perception

Clients who have an alteration in vision, smell, or taste can find it difficult to feed themselves or can find food unpalatable.

- Clients who have decreased vision might need assistance shopping for food on a regular basis, and with food preparation.
- Clients in a health care or long-term care facility might need help with tray setup and location of food on the tray.
- Clients who have an altered sense of smell have an altered sense of taste.
- Clients who smoke might have a diminished sense of smell.
- Clients receiving chemotherapy and other types of medications can experience taste alterations such as a metallic taste in their mouth, masking the real taste of food.
- Clients receiving radiation to the head and neck can experience altered or loss of taste (mouth blindness).

NURSING CARE
- Encourage the client who has decreased vision to consider shopping with a friend or family member, or have groceries delivered to the house. Qpcc
- Contact social services regarding availability of food or meal delivery to the client's home.
- Recommend to the client who has a food aversion to eat foods that are served cool, as they are typically less aromatic and are less likely to precipitate nausea.
- Suggest consuming foods that are spicy or tangy to compensate for the decreased sense of taste.
- Recommend sucking on hard candies, mints, or chewing gum to counteract an unusual taste in the mouth.
- Instruct the client to avoid ingestion of empty calories. If an increase in calories and fluid is desired, milkshakes, juice, and supplements are good options.

Impairment in swallowing

Clients who have neurologic disorders (Parkinson's disease, cerebral palsy, stroke) or had a surgical procedure done on their mouth, throat, epiglottis, or larynx can have difficulty managing food and swallowing without choking.

- Clients who have a neurologic disorder affecting the muscles in the mouth and throat are at risk for aspiration due to delayed swallowing and/or inadequate mastication.
- Clients who have a history of oral cancer might have had part of their lip, tongue, and/or soft palate removed. This significantly affects the ability to masticate and coordinate the development of a bolus of food prior to swallowing.
- The larynx and epiglottis prevent food from entering the trachea. Clients who have had partial or total removal of these can easily aspirate food and fluids, unless special precautions are taken.

NURSING CARE
- Continually monitor clients who are at risk for aspiration during meals, and have suction equipment immediately available. Qs
- Consult a dietitian regarding an appropriate diet for the client. The National Dysphagia diet includes three levels of solid textures.
  - Level 1: Pureed
  - Level 2: Mechanically altered
  - Level 3: Advanced

- Thicken thin fluids with a commercial thickener to the prescribed consistency of thin, nectar-like, honey-like, or spoon-thick.
- Allow adequate time for assisting the client who has dysphagia to eat. Have the client rest before meals.
- Teach clients who aspirate easily due to surgical alteration of their throat or upper tracheal structures to tuck their chins when swallowing. Arching the tongue in the back of the throat can help close off the trachea.

Mechanical fixation of the jaw

Disorders of the jaw requiring surgery include facial trauma and reconstruction.

- After fractured bones are realigned, the client's upper and lower jaw might be wired together.
- The jaw can be immobilized for several weeks.
- The client is generally placed on a liquid diet during this period.

NURSING CARE
- Encourage the intake of fluids.
- Help the client determine where to insert a straw through the space between the jaws.
- Work with the dietitian to develop a liquid meal plan that includes the necessary nutrients. Qtc

Lack of knowledge and misinformation about nutrition

Clients can be subject to overnutrition, undernutrition, and the ingestion of an inadequate intake of essential nutrients.

- Clients might not have basic knowledge about nutrition.
- Information about nutrition can be confusing or misleading.
- Clients can be drawn to fad diets (which are generally unhealthy) because quick results are promised.
- Clients can be misled by false advertising.

NURSING CARE
- Encourage clients to use dietary guidelines available from government and health associations (MyPlate [www.choosemyplate.gov], American Heart Association, Office of Disease Prevention and Health Promotion Dietary Guidelines [https://health.gov/dietaryguidelines]). Qebp
- Assist clients in locating community resources that provide education on nutrition.
- Assess dietary intake.
- Instruct clients on how to read nutrition fact labels.
- Encourage the client to keep a journal of dietary intake.
- Provide clients with information on foods that are healthy and portion sizes.
- Warn clients that advertisements can be fraudulent.

Medical conditions

- Clients who have medical conditions (cancer, COPD, burns, severe trauma, or HIV/AIDS) are at increased risk for malnutrition due to anorexia, nausea, or stomatitis related to treatments, increased metabolic demands, or the inability to consume a diet.
- Clients who are undergoing diagnostic testing that require NPO status are potentially at risk.
- Clients who have comorbidities resulting in polypharmacy are at risk for malnutrition and medication nutrient interactions.

NURSING CARE

- Monitor diet prescriptions and laboratory results, particularly for clients who are NPO or are receiving clear or full liquid diets for more than 24 hr. Refer the client to a dietitian for a complete evaluation of nutritional status. Q_{TC}
- Monitor clients who have comorbidities for interactions between medications and nutrition. Refer the client to a pharmacist for a thorough evaluation of medication interactions and the impact upon nutritional intake.
- Offer several small meals or snacks through the day instead of three large meals if the client cannot tolerate large amounts at once.
- Provide oral care prior to and following meals.
- Discourage the use of alcohol-based mouthwashes for clients who have stomatitis.
- Provide liquid supplements between meals to increase nutrient intake.

Active Learning Scenario

A nurse is providing dietary teaching for a client who requests assistance for weight loss. The client states, "I've tried several fad diets but they don't work for me." Use the ATI Active Learning Template: Basic Concept to complete this item to include the following sections.

UNDERLYING PRINCIPLES: Identify the client's barrier to nutrition.

NURSING INTERVENTIONS: Identify at least four interventions to address this client's barrier to nutrition and to promote healthy weight loss.

Application Exercises

1. A nurse is caring for several clients in an extended care facility. Which of the following clients is the highest priority to observe during meals?

   A. A client who has decreased vision

   B. A client who has Parkinson's disease

   C. A client who has poor dentition

   D. A client who has anorexia

2. A nurse is planning care for a client who is receiving treatment for malnutrition. The client is scheduled for discharge to their home where they live alone. Which of the following actions should the nurse include in the plan of care? (Select all that apply.)

   A. Consult social services to arrange home meal delivery.

   B. Encourage the client to purchase nonperishable boxed meals.

   C. Advise the client to purchase frozen fruits and vegetables.

   D. Recommend drinking a supplement between meals.

   E. Educate the client on how to read nutrition labels.

3. A nurse is providing teaching for a client who has a new diagnosis of hypertension and a prescription for a low-sodium diet. Which of the following client statements indicate an understanding of the teaching? (Select all that apply.)

   A. "I should select organic canned vegetables."

   B. "I need to read food labels when grocery shopping."

   C. "I will stop eating frozen dinners for lunch at work."

   D. "I know that deli meats are usually high in sodium."

   E. "I can refer to the American Heart Association's website for dietary guidelines."

4. A nurse is caring for a client who is transitioning to an oral diet following a partial laryngectomy. Which of the following actions should the nurse take to reduce the client's risk for aspiration?

   A. Request to have the client's oral medications provided in liquid form.

   B. Instruct the client to follow each bite of food with a drink of water.

   C. Encourage the client to tuck the chin when swallowing.

   D. Consult the dietitian about providing the client with a thin liquid diet.

5. A nurse is planning care for a client who has mechanical fixation of the jaw following a motorcycle crash. Which of the following actions should the nurse include in the plan of care? (Select all that apply.)

   A. Thicken liquids to honey consistency.

   B. Educate the client about the use of a nasogastric tube.

   C. Assist the client to use a straw to drink liquids.

   D. Ensure that the client receives ground meats.

   E. Encourage intake of fluids between meals.

Application Exercises Key

1. A. Observation of a client who has decreased vision is necessary to evaluate the client's need for assistance. However, this client is not the highest priority to observe during meals.
   B. **CORRECT:** A client who has Parkinson's disease is at risk for aspiration. Due to this safety risk, this client is the highest priority to observe during meals.
   C. Observation of a client who has poor dentition is necessary to evaluate the client's need for assistance or a modified diet. However, this client is not the highest priority to observe during meals.
   D. Observation of a client who has anorexia is necessary to evaluate the client's intake. However, this client is not the highest priority to observe during meals.

   Ⓝ *NCLEX® Connection: Safety and Infection Control, Accident/Error/Injury Prevention*

2. A. **CORRECT:** Consult social services to arrange home meal delivery to promote adequate nutrition.
   B. Boxed foods are usually high in calories and salt and are therefore not recommended to promote adequate nutrition.
   C. **CORRECT:** Advise the client to purchase frozen fruits and vegetables to promote adequate nutrition.
   D. **CORRECT:** Recommend a supplement between meals to promote adequate nutrition.
   E. **CORRECT:** Educate the client on how to read food labels to promote adequate nutrition.

   Ⓝ *NCLEX® Connection: Physiological Adaptation, Illness Management*

3. A. Canned foods, even if organic, are usually high in sodium and are therefore a poor choice for a client on a sodium-restricted diet.
   B. **CORRECT:** Reading food labels provides the client with information about the food's sodium content.
   C. **CORRECT:** Frozen dinners are usually high in sodium and are therefore a poor choice for a client on a sodium-restricted diet.
   D. **CORRECT:** Deli meats are usually high in sodium and are therefore a poor choice for a client on a sodium-restricted diet.
   E. **CORRECT:** The American Heart Association is a recommended health association for continued client education on dietary guidelines related to cardiac disorders such as hypertension.

   Ⓝ *NCLEX® Connection: Physiological Adaptation, Illness Management*

4. A. Providing medications in liquid form does not decrease the risk for aspiration.
   B. Drinking thin liquids, such as water, increases the risk for aspiration.
   C. **CORRECT:** Tucking the chin when swallowing helps to close off the trachea and reduces the risk for aspiration.
   D. Thick, rather than thin, liquids help reduce the risk for aspiration.

   Ⓝ *NCLEX® Connection: Reduction of Risk Potential, Potential for Complications of Diagnostic Tests/Treatments/Procedures*

5. A. Mechanical fixation of the jaw does not cause dysphagia. It is not necessary to thicken the client's liquids.
   B. Mechanical fixation of the jaw does not indicate the need for a nasogastric tube.
   C. **CORRECT:** Recommend the use of a straw to drink liquids. Help the client determine where to insert the straw through the space between the jaws.
   D. Mechanical fixation of the jaw indicates the need for a liquid diet rather than ground meats.
   E. **CORRECT:** The client who has a mechanical fixation of the jaw will have the jaws wired shut and is only able to consume liquids. Encourage supplemental and nutrient-rich liquids to maintain adequate hydration and nutrition.

   Ⓝ *NCLEX® Connection: Basic Care and Comfort, Nutrition and Oral Hydration*

Active Learning Scenario Key

Using the ATI Active Learning Template: Basic Concept

UNDERLYING PRINCIPLES: The client's barrier to nutrition is lack of knowledge and misinformation about nutrition. This barrier must be acknowledged to promote adequate nutrition.

NURSING INTERVENTIONS
- Encourage the client to use dietary guidelines such as MyPlate.
- Assist the client in locating community resources that provide education and nutrition to support healthy nutrition and weight loss.
- Advise the client that fad diets are generally unhealthy and often include false advertising.
- Perform an assessment of dietary intake.
- Encourage the client to keep a journal of dietary intake.
- Provide the client with information on healthy foods and portion sizes.

Ⓝ *NCLEX® Connection: Health Promotion and Maintenance, Health Promotion/Disease Prevention*

Cardiovascular and Hematologic Disorders

Nurses must have an awareness of nutritional needs for clients who have cardiovascular and hematologic disorders. It is important to explore dietary needs with the client and recommend modifications related to the disease process. Understanding the role of primary and secondary prevention is essential to successful treatment.

Cardiovascular diseases are the leading cause of death in the U.S. Coronary heart disease (CHD) is the single leading cause of death.

ASSESSMENT/DATA COLLECTION

Coronary heart disease

Hypercholesterolemia leads to atherosclerosis, a process of damage and cholesterol deposits on the blood vessels of the heart. Atherosclerosis is the cause of many cardiovascular disease complications (myocardial infarction, kidney failure, ischemic strokes).

- High-density lipoprotein (HDL) cholesterol is "good" cholesterol because it removes cholesterol from the body tissue and takes it to the liver. Levels greater than or equal to 60 mg/dL for males and 70 mg/dL or greater for females provide some protection against heart disease.
- Low-density lipoprotein (LDL) cholesterol is "bad" cholesterol because it transports cholesterol out of the liver and into the circulatory system, where it can form plaques on the coronary artery walls. The optimal range for LDL is less than 130 mg/dL.
- Optimal total cholesterol level is less than 200 mg/dL. Q_{EBP}

RISK FACTORS
- NON-MODIFIABLE: increasing age, male sex, family history of early CHD
- MODIFIABLE: high LDL cholesterol, low HDL cholesterol, consuming a diet high in saturated fat, hypertension, diabetes mellitus, metabolic syndrome, obesity, sedentary lifestyle, nicotine use disorder

Metabolic syndrome

The presence of three of the five following risk factors.
- Abdominal obesity
  - MALES: greater than or equal to 40-inch waist
  - FEMALES: greater than or equal to 35-inch waist
  - For Asian and non-European clients who have lived predominantly outside the U.S., use population- or country-specific definitions.
- Triglycerides greater than or equal to 150 mg/dL or taking medications to treat high triglyceride levels
- Low HDL or taking medications to lower HDL-C
  - MALES: less than or equal to 40 mg/dL
  - FEMALES: less than or equal to 50 mg/dL
- Increased blood pressure or taking an antihypertensive medication
  - Systolic greater than or equal to 130 mm/Hg
  - Diastolic greater than or equal to 85 mm/Hg
- Fasting blood glucose greater than or equal to 100 mg/dL or taking medication to control blood glucose levels

ANEMIAS

Iron deficiency anemia

RISK FACTORS
- Blood loss, deficient iron intake from diet, alcohol use disorder, malabsorption syndromes, gastrectomy
- Metabolic increase caused by pregnancy, adolescence, infection

MANIFESTATIONS
- Fatigue
- Lethargy
- Pallor of nail beds
- Intolerance to cold
- Headache
- Tachycardia

> ! Children who have low iron intake can experience short attention spans and display poor intellectual performance before anemia begins.

Vitamin B$_{12}$ deficiency anemia (macrocytic)

RISK FACTORS: Lack of meat or dairy consumption, small bowel resection, chronic diarrhea, diverticula, tapeworm, excess of intestinal bacteria

MANIFESTATIONS
- Pallor
- Jaundice
- Weakness
- Fatigue

GASTROINTESTINAL FINDINGS
- Glossitis (inflamed tongue)
- Anorexia
- Indigestion
- Weight loss

NEUROLOGIC FINDINGS
- Decreased concentration
- Paresthesia (numbness) of hands and feet
- Decreased proprioception (sense of body position)
- Poor muscle coordination
- Increasing irritability
- Delirium

Folic acid deficiency anemia

RISK FACTORS: Poor nutritional intake of foods containing folic acid (green leafy vegetables, citrus fruits, dried bean, nuts), malabsorption syndromes (Crohn's disease), certain medications (anticonvulsants and oral contraceptives)

MANIFESTATIONS
- Fatigue
- Pallor
- Glossitis
- Irritability
- Diarrhea

> Findings of folic acid deficiency anemia mimic those for vitamin B_{12} deficiency anemia except for the neurologic manifestations.

NUTRITIONAL GUIDELINES AND NURSING INTERVENTIONS

Coronary heart disease

PREVENTATIVE NUTRITION
- Consuming a diet that is limited in trans fats, saturated fats, and cholesterol can reduce the risk of developing CHD. The Therapeutic Lifestyle Change (TLC) diet is designed to be a user-friendly eating guide to encourage dietary changes.
- Daily cholesterol intake should be less than 200 mg.
- Conservative use of red wine can reduce the risk of developing CHD.
- Increasing fiber and carbohydrate intake, avoiding saturated fat, and decreasing red meat consumption can decrease the risk for developing CHD.
- Increased intake of omega-3 fatty acids found in fish, flaxseed, soy beans, canola, and walnuts reduces the risk of coronary artery disease.
- Homocysteine is an amino acid. Elevated homocysteine levels can increase the risk of developing CHD. Deficiencies in folate and vitamins B_6 and B_{12} increase homocysteine levels.

THERAPEUTIC NUTRITION
- Secondary prevention efforts for CHD are focused on lifestyle changes that lower LDL. These include a diet low in cholesterol and saturated fats, a diet high in fiber, exercise and weight management, and cessation of nicotine use.
- Daily cholesterol intake should be less than 200 mg/day. Saturated fat should be limited to less than 7% of daily caloric intake.
- To lower cholesterol and saturated fats, instruct the client to do the following.
  - Trim visible fat from meats.
  - Limit red meats and choose lean meats (turkey, chicken).
  - Remove the skin from meats.
  - Broil, bake, grill, or steam foods. Avoid frying foods.
  - Use low-fat or nonfat milk, cheese, and yogurt.
  - Use spices in place of butter or salt to season foods.
  - Use liquid oils (olive or canola) in place of oils that are high in saturated fat (lard, butter).
  - Avoid trans fat, which increases LDL. Partially hydrogenated products contain trans fat.
  - Increase consumption of oily fish (tuna, salmon, herring).
  - Read labels.
- Encourage the client to consume a high-fiber diet.
  - Soluble fiber lowers LDL.
  - Oats, beans, fruits, vegetables, whole grains, barley, and flaxseed are good sources of fiber.
- Encourage the client to exercise.
  - Instruct the client regarding practical methods for increasing physical activity. (Encourage the client to take the stairs rather than the elevator.)
  - Provide the client with references for local exercise facilities.
- Instruct the client to stop all use of tobacco products.
- The recommended lifestyle changes represent a significant change for many clients. ○PCC
  - Provide support to the client and family.
  - Encourage the client's family to participate in the changes to ease the transition for the client.
  - Explain why the diet is important.
  - Aid the client in developing a diet that is complementary to personal food preferences and lifestyle. A food diary can be helpful.
  - Instruct the client that occasional deviations from the diet are reasonable.

Hypertension

- Hypertension is a significant risk factor for developing CHD, myocardial infarction, kidney disease, and stroke.
- Hypertension is a sustained elevation in blood pressure greater than or equal to 130/80 mm Hg.

RISK FACTORS FOR PRIMARY HYPERTENSION: family history, hyperlipidemia, smoking, obesity, physical inactivity, high sodium intake, low potassium intake, excessive alcohol consumption, stress, and aging. African-American people have the highest prevalence of hypertension. A client's risk of hypertension increases after menopause.

THERAPEUTIC NUTRITION
- The Dietary Approaches to Stopping Hypertension (DASH) diet is a low-sodium, high-potassium, high-calcium diet that has proven to lower blood pressure (systolic and diastolic) and cholesterol.
  - Decrease sodium intake (initially a daily intake of less than 2,300 mg is recommended, and should gradually be decreased to 1,500 mg for maximum benefit).
  - Foods high in sodium include canned soups and sauces, potato chips, pretzels, smoked meats, seasonings, and processed foods.
  - Include low-fat dairy products to promote calcium intake.
  - Include fruits and vegetables rich in potassium (apricots, bananas, tomatoes, potatoes).
- Limit alcohol intake.
- Encourage the client to read labels and educate the client about appropriate food choices.
- Other lifestyle changes include exercising, weight loss, and smoking cessation.

Heart failure

Heart failure is characterized by the inability of the heart to maintain adequate blood flow throughout the circulatory system. It results in excess sodium and fluid retention, and edema.

RISK FACTORS: CHD, arrhythmias, previous MI, valve disorders, hypertension, obesity, diabetes, metabolic syndrome

THERAPEUTIC NUTRITION
- Reduce sodium intake to less than 3,000 mg per day for mild-to-moderate heart failure and less than 2,000 mg/day for severe heart failure.
- Monitor fluid intake (and possibly restrict 2 L/day).
- Increase protein intake to 1.12 g/kg.
- Use small, frequent meals that are soft, easy-to-chew foods.

Myocardial infarction

- A myocardial infarction (MI) occurs when there is an inadequate supply of oxygen to the myocardium.
- After an MI, it is necessary to reduce the myocardial oxygen demands related to metabolic activity.
- Risk factors are the same as for CHD.

THERAPEUTIC NUTRITION
- A liquid diet is best for the first 24 hr after the infarction.
- Caffeine should be avoided because it stimulates the heart and increases heart rate.
- Small, frequent meals are indicated.
- Counsel the client about recommendations for a heart-healthy diet.

Anemia

Anemia results from either a reduction in the number of red blood cells (RBCs) or in hemoglobin, the oxygen-carrying component of blood. Anemia can result from a decrease in RBC production, an increase in RBC destruction, or a loss of blood.
- The body requires iron, vitamin B_{12}, and folic acid to produce red blood cells.
- Iron deficiency anemia is the most common nutritional disorder in the world. It affects approximately 10% of the U.S. population, especially older infants, toddlers, adolescent females, and pregnant clients.
- From childhood until adolescence, iron intake tends to be marginal.
- Pernicious anemia is the most common form of vitamin B_{12} deficiency. It is caused by lack of intrinsic factor, a protein that helps the body absorb vitamin B_{12}.

SOURCES OF IRON
- Meat
- Fish
- Poultry
- Tofu
- Dried peas and beans
- Whole grains
- Dried fruit
- Iron-fortified foods
  - Infant formula (alternative or supplement to breastfeeding)
  - Infant cereal (usually the first food introduced to infants)
  - Ready-to-eat cereals

VITAMIN C: Facilitates the absorption of iron (promote consumption).

! Medicinal iron toxicity is the leading cause of accidental poisoning in small children and can lead to acute iron toxicity. Qs

NATURAL SOURCES OF VITAMIN B_{12}
- Fish
- Meat
- Poultry
- Eggs
- Milk

People older than 50 years are urged to consume most of their vitamin B_{12} requirement from supplements or fortified food.

People who follow a vegan diet need supplemental B_{12}.

FOLIC ACID SOURCES
- Green leafy vegetables
- Dried peas and beans
- Seeds
- Orange juice
- Cereals and breads fortified with folic acid

If the client is unable to obtain an adequate supply of folic acid, supplementation can be necessary.

Application Exercises

1. A nurse is teaching a client about dietary recommendations to lower high blood pressure. Which of the following statements by the client indicates understanding?

   A. "My daily sodium consumption should be 3,000 milligrams."

   B. "I should consume foods low in potassium."

   C. "My limit is three cigarettes a day."

   D. "I should consume low-fat dairy products."

2. A nurse is teaching a client about high-fiber foods that can assist in lowering LDL. Which of the following foods should the nurse include? (Select all that apply.)

   A. Beans

   B. Cheese

   C. Whole grains

   D. Broccoli

   E. Yogurt

3. A community health nurse is assessing a client who reports numbness of the hands and feet for the past 2 weeks. This finding is associated with which of the following nutritional deficiencies?

   A. Folic acid

   B. Potassium

   C. Vitamin B_{12}

   D. Iron

4. A nurse is reviewing a client health record that includes a report of abdominal obesity and laboratory findings of elevated blood glucose and elevated triglycerides. These findings meet the criteria of which of the following conditions?

   A. Anemia

   B. Metabolic syndrome

   C. Heart failure

   D. Hypertension

5. A nurse is providing teaching to a client who has vitamin B_{12} deficiency. Which of the following foods should the nurse instruct the client to consume? (Select all that apply.)

   A. Meat

   B. Flaxseed

   C. Beans

   D. Eggs

   E. Milk

Active Learning Scenario

A nurse is providing teaching to a client who has hypertension. What should the nurse include in the teaching? Use the ATI Active Learning Template: System Disorder to complete this item to include the following sections.

ALTERATION IN HEALTH (DIAGNOSIS)

CLIENT EDUCATION: Describe the Dietary Approaches to Stopping Hypertension (DASH) diet and four nutrition teaching points to include.

Application Exercises Key

1. A. Daily sodium consumption should be 2,300 mg or less. This assists with lowering systolic and diastolic blood pressures as well as cholesterol.
   B. Foods high in potassium should be encouraged. This assists with lowering systolic and diastolic blood pressures as well as cholesterol.
   C. Smoking cessation should be encouraged. Smoking can increase blood pressure and should be avoided.
   D. **CORRECT:** Low-fat dairy products should be encouraged. They promote calcium intake and assist with lowering systolic and diastolic blood pressures as well as cholesterol.

   Ⓝ *NCLEX® Connection: Basic Care and Comfort, Nutrition and Oral Hydration*

2. A. **CORRECT:** Beans are high in fiber and should be included in the teaching.
   B. Cheese is high in calcium and should not be included in the teaching.
   C. **CORRECT:** Whole grains are high in fiber and should be included in the teaching.
   D. **CORRECT:** Broccoli is high in fiber and should be included in the teaching.
   E. Yogurt is high in calcium and should not be included in the teaching.

   Ⓝ *NCLEX® Connection: Basic Care and Comfort, Nutrition and Oral Hydration*

3. A. Pallor, glossitis, and gastrointestinal distress are manifestations associated with folic acid deficiency.
   B. Irritability, decreased respirations, muscle weakness, and gastrointestinal distress are manifestations associated with hypokalemia.
   C. **CORRECT:** Numbness of the hands and feet are manifestations associated with vitamin B$_{12}$ deficiency.
   D. Fatigue, lethargy, pallor of nail beds, and intolerance to cold are manifestations associated with iron deficiency anemia.

   Ⓝ *NCLEX® Connection: Basic Care and Comfort, Nutrition and Oral Hydration*

4. A. Fatigue, lethargy, pallor of nail beds, and intolerance to cold are manifestations associated with anemia.
   B. **CORRECT:** Weight gain in the abdomen, elevated blood glucose, and elevated triglycerides are manifestations associated with metabolic syndrome.
   C. Shortness of breath, fluid retention, and fatigue are manifestations associated with heart failure.
   D. Headaches, tiredness, and dizziness are manifestations associated with hypertension.

   Ⓝ *NCLEX® Connection: Basic Care and Comfort, Nutrition and Oral Hydration*

5. A. **CORRECT:** Meat is a food source that is high in vitamin B$_{12}$.
   B. Flaxseed is a good source of fiber.
   C. Beans are a good source of folic acid.
   D. **CORRECT:** Eggs are a food source that is high in vitamin B$_{12}$.
   E. **CORRECT:** Milk is a food source that is high in vitamin B$_{12}$.

   Ⓝ *NCLEX® Connection: Basic Care and Comfort, Nutrition and Oral Hydration*

Active Learning Scenario Key

Using the ATI Active Learning Template: System Disorder

ALTERATION IN HEALTH (DIAGNOSIS): Hypertension is a sustained elevation in blood pressure greater than or equal to 140/90 mm Hg in clients less than age 60 and 150/90 mm Hg in those older than 60.

CLIENT EDUCATION
- The DASH diet is a low-sodium, high-potassium, high-calcium diet that has been proven to lower blood pressure and cholesterol.
- Lower sodium intake (daily intake of less than 2,300 mg) is recommended.
- Foods high in sodium include canned soups and sauces, potato chips, pretzels, smoked meats, seasonings, and processed foods.
- Include low-fat dairy products to promote calcium intake.
- Include fruits and vegetables rich in potassium (apricots, bananas, tomatoes, potatoes).
- Limit alcohol intake.

Ⓝ *NCLEX® Connection: Physiological Adaptation, Illness Management*

UNIT 3   ALTERATIONS IN NUTRITION

CHAPTER 13 *Gastrointestinal Disorders*

Nurses must gain an awareness of nutritional needs for clients who have gastrointestinal (GI) disorders. It is important to explore dietary needs with the client and recommend modifications in relationship to the disease process. Understanding the role of primary and secondary prevention is essential to successful treatment.

Nutrition therapy for gastrointestinal disorders is generally aimed at minimizing or preventing manifestations. In some conditions (celiac disease), nutrition is the only treatment. For some GI disorders, nutrition therapy is the foundation of treatment.

ASSESSMENT/DATA COLLECTION

- Determine whether the client is experiencing any of the following.
  - Difficulty chewing or swallowing
  - Nausea, vomiting, or diarrhea
  - Bloating, excessive flatus, occult blood, steatorrhea, abdominal pain or cramping, abdominal distention, pale, sticky bowel movements
  - Changes in weight, eating patterns, or bowel habits
- Determine whether the client uses the following.
  - Tobacco
  - Alcohol
  - Caffeine
  - Over-the-counter medications to treat GI conditions (many can have GI complications or be contraindicated with GI conditions)
  - Nutritional supplements
  - Herbal supplements for GI conditions or other problems (some clients do not consider them to be medications, so they do not mention them to the provider)

NUTRITIONAL GUIDELINES AND NURSING INTERVENTIONS

General gastrointestinal considerations

- Monitor gastrointestinal parameters.
  - Weight and weight changes
  - Laboratory values
  - Elimination patterns
  - I&O
- Low-fiber diets avoid foods that are high in residue content (whole-grain breads and cereals, raw fruits and vegetables).
  - Diets low in fiber reduce the frequency and volume of fecal output and slow transit time of food through the digestive tract.
  - Low-fiber diets are used short-term for clients who have diarrhea or malabsorption syndromes.
- High-fiber diets focus on foods containing more than 5 g of fiber per serving. A diet high in fiber helps:
  - Increase stool bulk.
  - Stimulate peristalsis.
  - Prevent constipation.
  - Protect against colon cancer.

Nausea and vomiting

- Potential causes of nausea and vomiting include decreased gastric acid secretion; decreased gastrointestinal motility; allergy to food(s); bacterial or viral infection; increased intracranial pressure; liver, pancreatic, and gall bladder disorders; and adverse effects of some medications.
- The underlying cause of nausea and vomiting should be investigated. Assessing the appearance of the emesis will aid in diagnosis and treatment (coffee-ground emesis indicates the presence of blood; pale green indicates bile).
- Once manifestations subside, begin with clear liquids followed by full liquids, and advance the diet as tolerated.
- Easy-to-digest, low-fat carbohydrate foods (crackers, toast, oatmeal, pretzels, plain bread, bland fruit) are usually well-tolerated.

NURSING ACTIONS
- Promote good oral hygiene with tooth brushing, mouth swabs, mouthwash, and ice chips.
- Elevate the head of the bed.
- Serve foods at room temperature or chilled.

CLIENT EDUCATION
- Avoid hot and spicy foods.
- Avoid liquids with meals, as they promote a feeling of fullness.
- Avoid high-fat foods if they contribute to nausea because they are difficult to digest.

Anorexia

- Anorexia is defined as a lack of appetite. It is a common finding for numerous physical conditions and is an adverse effect of certain medications. It is not the same as anorexia nervosa.
- Anorexia can lead to decreased nutritional intake and subsequent protein and calorie deficits.

NURSING ACTIONS
- Decrease stress at meal times.
- Collect data regarding adverse effects of medications.
- Administer medications to stimulate appetite.
- Assess and modify environment for unpleasant odors.
- Remove items that cause a decrease in appetite (soiled linens, garbage, emesis basins, bedpans, used tissues, clutter).
- Assess and manage anxiety and depression.
- Provide small, frequent meals and avoid high-fat foods to help maximize intake. Beverages should be held at least 30 min before and after meals to prevent the client from feeling full before adequate intake of calories from food.
- Provide liquid supplements between meals to improve protein and calorie intake.
- Ensure that meals appear appealing. Serve larger meals early in the day.
- Assess for changes in bowel status (increased gastric emptying, constipation, diarrhea).
- Position to increase gastric motility.
- Provide mouth care before and after meals.

Constipation

- Clients who have constipation have difficult or infrequent passage of stools, which can be hard and dry.
- Causes include irregular bowel habits, psychogenic factors, inactivity, chronic laxative use, obstruction, medications, GI disorders (irritable bowel syndrome [IBS]), pregnancy, or secondary to genital/rectal trauma (sexual abuse or childbirth), and inadequate consumption of fiber and fluid.
- Encourage exercise and a diet high in fiber (25 g/day for females and 38 g/day for males), and promote adequate fluid intake to help alleviate constipation.
- If caused by medication, a change in the medication might be necessary.

NURSING ACTIONS
- Determine onset and duration of past and present elimination patterns, what is normal for the client, activity levels, occupation, dietary intake, and stress levels.
- Collect data about past medical and surgical history, medication use (OTC, herbal supplements, laxatives, enemas, and prescriptions), presence of rectal pressure or fullness, and abdominal pain.
- Encourage client to gradually increase daily intake of fiber.

CLIENT EDUCATION
- Increase fluid intake to 64 oz/day unless contraindicated.
- An increase in fiber intake is the preferred treatment for constipation. Avoid chronic use of laxatives.

Diarrhea

- Diarrhea can cause significant losses of potassium, sodium, and fluid, as well as nutritional complications.
- Common causes of diarrhea include emotional and physical stress, gastrointestinal disorders, malabsorption disorders, infections, and certain medications.
- Low-fiber diets might be recommended on a short-term basis to decrease bowel stimulation.
- Nutrition therapy varies with the severity and duration of diarrhea. A liberal fluid intake to replace losses is needed.

Dysphagia

- Dysphagia is an alteration in the client's ability to swallow.
- Causes include obstruction, inflammation, and certain neurologic disorders.
- Modifying the texture of foods and the consistency of liquids can enable the client to achieve proper nutrition.
- Dry mouth can contribute to dysphagia. Evaluate medications being taken to determine if this is a potential adverse effect.
- Clients who have dysphagia should be referred to a speech therapist for evaluation.
- Dietary modifications are based on the specific swallowing limitations experienced by the client.
- Nutritional supplements are beneficial if nutritional intake is deemed inadequate.

NURSING ACTIONS
- Clients who have dysphagia are at an increased risk of aspiration. Place the client in an upright or high-Fowler's position to facilitate swallowing. Qs
- Provide oral care prior to eating to enhance the client's sense of taste.
- Allow adequate time for eating, use adaptive eating devices, and encourage small bites and thorough chewing.

CLIENT EDUCATION
- Pills should be taken with at least 8 oz of fluid (can be thickened) to prevent medication from remaining in the esophagus.
- Avoid thin liquids and sticky foods.

Dumping syndrome

Normally, the stomach controls the rate in which nutrients enter the small intestine. When a portion of the stomach is surgically removed, the contents of the stomach are rapidly emptied into the small intestine, causing dumping syndrome.
- Early manifestations typically occur 10 to 20 min after eating. Early manifestations include a sensation of fullness, abdominal cramping, nausea, diarrhea, and vasomotor manifestations (faintness, syncope, diaphoresis, tachycardia, hypotension, flushing).
- Late manifestations occur 1 to 3 hr after eating. Late manifestations include diaphoresis, weakness, tremors, anxiety, nausea, and hunger.
- Manifestations resolve after intestine is emptied. However, there is a rapid rise in blood glucose and increase in insulin levels immediately after the intestine empties. This leads to hypoglycemia.

NURSING ACTIONS

- Monitor clients receiving enteral tube feedings and report manifestations of dumping syndrome to the provider.
- Monitor the client for vitamin and mineral deficits (iron and vitamin B_{12}).

CLIENT EDUCATION

- Consume small, frequent meals.
- Consume protein and fat at each meal.
- Avoid food that contains concentrated sugars and restrict lactose intake.
- Plan to consume liquids 1 hr after meals or between meals (no sooner than 30 min after eating).
- Lie down after meals to delay gastric emptying. If reflux is a problem, try a reclining position.

Gastroesophageal reflux disease

- Gastroesophageal reflux disease (GERD) occurs as the result of the abnormal reflux of gastric secretions up the esophagus. This leads to indigestion and heartburn.
- Factors that contribute to GERD include hiatal hernia, obesity, pregnancy, smoking, some medications, and genetics.
- Long-term GERD can cause serious complications, including adenocarcinoma of the esophagus and Barrett's esophagus.
- Manifestations include heartburn, retrosternal burning, painful swallowing, dyspepsia, regurgitation, coughing, hoarseness, and epigastric pain. Pain can be mistaken for a myocardial infarction.

CLIENT EDUCATION

- Avoid situations that lead to increased abdominal pressure, such as wearing tight fitting clothing.
- Avoid eating for 3 hr before lying down.
- Elevate the body on pillows instead of lying flat and avoid large meals and bedtime snacks.
- Attempt weight loss if overweight or obese.
- Avoid trigger foods (citrus fruits and juices, spicy foods, carbonated beverages).
- Avoid items that reduce lower esophageal sphincter pressure (fatty foods, caffeine, chocolate, alcohol, cigarette smoke, all nicotine products, peppermint and spearmint flavors).

Acute and chronic gastritis

- Gastritis is characterized by inflammation of the gastric mucosa. The gastric mucosa is congested with blood and fluid, becoming inflamed. There is a decrease in acid produced and an overabundance of mucus. Superficial ulcers occur, sometimes leading to hemorrhages.
- Acute gastritis occurs with excessive use of NSAIDs, bile reflux, ingestion of a strong acid or alkali substance, as a complication of radiation therapy, or as a complication of trauma (burns; food poisoning; severe infection; liver, kidney, or respiratory failure; major surgery).
- Chronic gastritis occurs in the presence of ulcers (benign or malignant), *Helicobacter pylori*, autoimmune disorders (pernicious anemia), poor diet (excessive caffeine, excessive alcohol intake), medications (alendronate, perindopril), and reflux of pancreatic secretions and bile into stomach.

- Manifestations include abdominal pain or discomfort (can be relieved by eating), headache, lethargy, nausea, anorexia, hiccuping (lasting a few hours to days), heartburn after eating, belching, sour taste in mouth, vomiting, bleeding, and hematemesis (vomiting of blood).
- Acute recovery typically occurs in 1 day, but can take 2 to 3 days. The client should eat a bland diet when able to tolerate food. IV fluid replacement therapy is indicated if the condition persists.
- When the condition occurs due to ingestion of strong acids or alkalis, dilution and neutralization of the causal agent is needed. Avoid lavage and emetics due to potential perforation and esophageal damage. Qs

CHRONIC MANAGEMENT: Modify diet, reduce and manage stress, avoid alcohol and NSAIDs. If condition is persistent, the provider will prescribe an H_2 receptor antagonist (famotidine). QEBP

NURSING ACTIONS: Monitor for vitamin deficiency, especially of vitamin B_{12}.

CLIENT EDUCATION

- Avoid eating frequent meals and snacks, as they promote increased gastric acid secretion.
- Avoid alcohol, cigarette smoking, aspirin and other nonsteroidal anti-inflammatory drugs (NSAIDs), coffee, black pepper, spicy foods, and caffeine.

Peptic ulcer disease

- Peptic ulcer disease (PUD) is characterized by an erosion of the mucosal layer of the stomach or duodenum. This can be caused by a bacterial infection with *H. pylori* or the chronic use of NSAIDs (aspirin, ibuprofen).
- Some clients who have PUD do not experience manifestations. Others report dull, gnawing pain, burning sensation in the back or low midepigastric area, heartburn, constipation or diarrhea, sour taste in mouth, burping, nausea, vomiting, bloating, urea present in breath, and tarry stools. Eating can temporarily relieve pain. Anemia can occur due to blood loss.
- For PUD caused by *H. pylori*, the provider prescribes triple therapy (a combination of antibiotics and acid reducing medications) to be taken for 10 to 14 days.

CLIENT EDUCATION: Avoid coffee, alcohol, caffeine, aspirin and other NSAIDs, cigarette smoking, black pepper, and spicy foods.

Lactose intolerance

- Lactose intolerance results from an inadequate supply of lactase in the intestine, the enzyme that digests lactose.
- The enzyme that converts lactose into glucose, and galactose is absent or insufficient. Manifestations include distention, cramps, flatus, and osmotic diarrhea.
- Small amounts (4 to 6 oz) of milk taken during meals can be tolerated.
- Some dairy products (yogurt, aged cheeses) are low in lactate and can be better tolerated.

NURSING ACTIONS: Monitor for vitamin D and calcium deficiency.

NURSING ACTIONS

- Avoid or limit intake of foods high in lactose (milk, soft cheese, ice cream, cream soups, sour cream, puddings, coffee creamer).
- Ask the provider about the use of a lactase enzyme.

Ileostomies and colostomies

An ostomy is a surgically created opening on the surface of the abdomen from either the end of the small intestine (ileostomy) or from the colon (colostomy).

- Fluid and electrolyte maintenance is the primary concern for clients who have ileostomies and colostomies.
- The colon absorbs large amounts of fluid, sodium, and potassium.
- Nutrition therapy begins with liquids only and is slowly advanced based upon client tolerance.

NURSING ACTIONS: Provide emotional support to clients due to the risk of altered body image. Qpcc

CLIENT EDUCATION

- Consume a diet that is high in fluids (at least 1.9 to 2.4 L [64 to 80 oz] per day) and soluble fiber.
- Avoid foods that cause gas (beans, eggs, carbonated beverages), stomal blockage (nuts, raw carrots, popcorn), and foods that produce odor (eggs, fish, garlic).
- Increase intake of calories and protein to promote healing of the stoma site.

Diverticulosis and diverticulitis

Diverticula are pouches protruding through the muscle of the intestinal wall, usually from increased intraluminal pressure. They occur anywhere in the colon, but usually in the sigmoid colon. Unless infection occurs, diverticula cause no problems.

- Diverticulosis is a condition characterized by the presence of diverticula.
- Diverticulitis is inflammation that occurs when fecal matter becomes trapped in the diverticula.
- Manifestations of diverticulitis include abdominal pain, nausea, vomiting, constipation or diarrhea, and fever, accompanied by chills and tachycardia.
- The client receives antibiotics, anticholinergics, and analgesics. Clients who have severe manifestations are admitted to the hospital and dehydration is treated with IV therapy. Opioid analgesics are administered for pain. Complications (peritonitis, bowel obstruction, abscess) can warrant surgical intervention.
- A high-fiber diet can prevent diverticulosis and diverticulitis by producing stools that are easily passed, thus decreasing pressure within the colon.
- During acute diverticulitis, a clear liquid diet is prescribed until inflammation decreases, then a high-fiber, low-fat diet is indicated.
- Clients require instruction regarding diet adjustment based on the need for an acute intervention or preventive approach.

Inflammatory bowel disease (IBD)

- Crohn's disease (regional enteritis) and ulcerative colitis are chronic, inflammatory bowel diseases characterized by periods of exacerbation and remission.
- Manifestations include nausea, vomiting, abdominal cramps, fever, fatigue, anorexia, weight loss, steatorrhea, and low-grade fever.
- Nutrition therapy is focused on providing nutrients in forms that the client can tolerate.
- A low-residue, high-protein, high-calorie diet with vitamin and mineral supplementation is prescribed during exacerbation to minimize bowel stimulation. Fluid and electrolyte imbalances are corrected with IV fluids or oral replacement fluids.
- Enteral nutrition can be prescribed during exacerbations, especially if the client is reluctant to eat. Because parenteral nutrition is more costly with a relatively similar benefit, it is not used unless enteral nutrition is ineffective or contraindicated.
- When the client is not experiencing an exacerbation, the diet can be broadened based on the client's specific disease process and triggers.

Additional therapy
- Complementary therapies including vitamin C and herbs (flaxseed)
- Yoga, hypnosis, and breathing exercises
- Sedatives
- Antidiarrheal and antiperistaltic agents
- Aminosalicylate medications and corticosteroids to reduce inflammation
- Immunomodulators to alter the immune response and prevent relapse
- Surgery when other treatments are not effective

CLIENT EDUCATION: Avoid intake of substances that cause or exacerbate diarrhea, and avoid nicotine.

Cholecystitis

- Cholecystitis is characterized by inflammation of the gallbladder.
- The gallbladder stores and releases bile that aids in the digestion of fats.
- Manifestations include pain, tenderness, and rigidity in upper right abdomen. Pain can radiate to the right shoulder or midsternal area. Nausea, vomiting, and anorexia also can occur. If the gallbladder becomes filled with pus or becomes gangrenous, perforation can result.
- In clients who have large stones or inability to control the condition with diet modifications, surgery is required.
- Pancreatitis and liver involvement can result from uncontrolled cholecystitis.
- Fat intake should be limited to reduce stimulation of the gallbladder.
- The diet is individualized to the client's needs and tolerance.

Pancreatitis

- Pancreatitis is an inflammation of the pancreas, which can be acute or chronic. In 70% of the acute cases, alcohol use and gallstones are major causes. Chronic pancreatitis can result from acute pancreatitis that does not resolve.
- The pancreas is responsible for secreting enzymes needed to digest fats, carbohydrates, and proteins.
- Nutritional therapy for acute pancreatitis involves reducing pancreatic stimulation. The client is prescribed nothing by mouth (NPO), and a nasogastric tube is inserted to suction gastric contents.
- TPN can be used until oral intake is resumed.
- Nutritional therapy for chronic pancreatitis usually includes a low-fat, high-protein, and high-carbohydrate diet. It can include providing supplements of vitamin C and B-complex vitamins.

Liver disease

- The liver is involved in the metabolism of most nutrients.
- Disorders affecting the liver include cirrhosis, hepatitis, and cancer.
- Malnutrition is common with liver disease.
- Protein needs are increased to promote a positive nitrogen balance and prevent a breakdown of the body's protein stores.
- Carbohydrates are generally not restricted, as they are an important source of calories.
- Caloric requirements might need to be increased based on an evaluation of the client's stage of disease, weight, and general health status.
- Multivitamins (especially vitamins B, C, and K) and mineral supplements might be necessary.
- Alcohol, nicotine, and caffeine should be eliminated.

Celiac disease QPCC

- Celiac disease is also known as gluten-sensitive enteropathy, celiac sprue, and gluten intolerance.
- It is a chronic, inherited, genetic disorder with autoimmune characteristics. Clients who have celiac disease are unable to digest the protein gluten. They lack the digestive enzyme DPP-IV, which is required to break down the gluten into molecules small enough to be used by the body. In celiac disease, gluten is broken down into peptide strands instead of molecules. The body is not able to metabolize the peptides. If untreated, the client will suffer destruction of the villa and the walls of the small intestine. Celiac disease can go undiagnosed in both children and adults.
- Manifestations vary widely. Children who have celiac disease have diarrhea, steatorrhea, anemia, abdominal distention, impaired growth, lack of appetite, and fatigue. Typical manifestations in adults include diarrhea, abdominal pain, bloating, anemia, steatorrhea, and osteomalacia.

- Treatment for celiac disease is limited to avoiding gluten. However, eliminating gluten, which is found in wheat, rye and barley, is difficult because it is found in many prepared foods. Clients must read food labels carefully in order to adhere to a gluten-free diet. Some gluten-free products are unappealing to clients, and many are more expensive than other products. Prognosis is good for clients who adhere to a gluten-free diet.

NURSING ACTIONS

- Monitor for complications including bleeding (bruising) due to inadequate vitamin K intake, manifestations of anemias (iron, folate, vitamin B_{12}), and manifestations of osteoporosis.
- Collaborate with a dietitian to assist with food selection and label reading.

CLIENT EDUCATION

- Eat foods that are gluten-free (milk, cheese, rice, corn, eggs, potatoes, fruits, vegetables, fresh meats and fish, dried beans).
- Read labels on processed products. Gravy mixes, sauces, cold cuts, soups, and many other products have gluten as an ingredient.
- Read labels and research nonfood products (lipstick, communion wafers, vitamin supplements), which also can have gluten as an ingredient. QPCC

Bariatric surgery

This is considered the most effective treatment for managing obesity and related conditions. Benefits include reduction of diabetes mellitus, hypertension, dyslipidemia, and mortality rates as well as improved quality of life.

- Bariatric surgery works best in combination with diet and lifestyle changes. Nutritional counseling is essential. Protein intake of 60 g/day is required to prevent protein-calorie malnutrition.
- CLIENT EDUCATION: Dramatic changes in food intake and regular physical activity will be necessary for successful long-term weight control.

Adjustable gastric banding restricts stomach capacity to 15 to 30 mL with an inflatable band that encircles the uppermost portion of the stomach, similar to a belt to create an outlet that can be adjusted as needed.

- CLIENT EDUCATION
  - Diet will gradually increase from liquids to pureed to soft foods.
  - Chew foods thoroughly, slowly, and in small amounts.

Roux-en-Y gastric bypass: Ingested food bypasses 95% of the stomach, the duodenum, and a small portion of the proximal jejunum. Weight loss is achieved through malabsorption and dumping syndrome and the altering of the hormone ghrelin which decreases hunger.

- Possible postoperative complications include anastomotic leaks, internal hernias, GI bleeding, stomal stenosis, gallstones.
- Micronutrient deficiencies are common long term.

Sleeve gastrectomy is a procedure in which a longitudinal portion of the stomach is removed to create a "sleeve" effect. This reduces production of the hormone ghrelin, which decreases hunger.

Application Exercises

1. A nurse is teaching a client who is recovering from pancreatitis about following a low-fat diet. Which of the following foods should the nurse recommend? (Select all that apply.)
   - A. Ribeye steak
   - B. Oatmeal
   - C. Ice cream
   - D. Canned peaches
   - E. Pretzels

2. A nurse is teaching a client who has constipation about a high-fiber, low-fat diet. Which of the following food choices by the client indicates understanding of the teaching?
   - A. Peanut butter
   - B. Peeled apples
   - C. Hardboiled egg
   - D. Brown rice

3. A nurse is assessing a client who is postoperative from a gastric bypass and who just finished eating a meal. Which of the following findings are manifestations of dumping syndrome? (Select all that apply.)
   - A. Bradycardia
   - B. Dizziness
   - C. Dry skin
   - D. Hypotension
   - E. Diarrhea

4. A nurse is collecting data from a client who has peptic ulcer disease (PUD). Which of the following findings should the nurse expect? (Select all that apply.)
   - A. Steatorrhea
   - B. Anemia
   - C. Tarry stools
   - D. Epigastric pain
   - E. Swollen lymph nodes

5. A nurse is instructing a client who has celiac disease about foods to avoid. Which of the following foods should the nurse include in the teaching?
   - A. Potatoes
   - B. Graham crackers
   - C. Wild rice
   - D. Canned pears

Active Learning Scenario

A nurse is providing instructions to the guardian of a child who has lactose intolerance. What should the nurse include in the teaching? Use the ATI Active Learning Template: System Disorder to complete this item.

CLIENT EDUCATION
- Describe the underlying cause of lactose intolerance.
- Identify two manifestations of lactose intolerance.
- Identify three foods the child should limit or eliminate from their diet.

Application Exercises Key

1. A. Ribeye steak is not a low-fat food source.
   B. **CORRECT:** Oatmeal is a source of easily digested carbohydrate that is low in fat.
   C. Ice cream is not a low-fat food source.
   D. **CORRECT:** Canned peaches are a source of easily digested carbohydrate that is low in fat.
   E. **CORRECT:** Pretzels are a source of easily digested carbohydrate that is low in fat.

   Ⓝ *NCLEX® Connection: Basic Care and Comfort, Nutrition and Oral Hydration*

2. A. Peanut butter is high in fat.
   B. Unpeeled fruit is a better source of fiber.
   C. Egg yolk is high in fat.
   D. **CORRECT:** Brown rice is a good source of fiber and is low in fat.

   Ⓝ *NCLEX® Connection: Basic Care and Comfort, Elimination*

3. A. Tachycardia due to a decrease in circulating volume is a manifestation of dumping syndrome.
   B. **CORRECT:** When a portion of the stomach is no longer available to serve as a reservoir, a large amount of food is rapidly dumped into the small intestine, and fluid shifts from general circulation into the intestine. Dizziness occurs due to a decrease in circulating volume.
   C. Sweating is a manifestation of dumping syndrome.
   D. **CORRECT:** Hypotension occurs due to a decrease in circulating volume.
   E. **CORRECT:** Diarrhea from increased peristalsis is a manifestation of dumping syndrome.

   Ⓝ *NCLEX® Connection: Basic Care and Comfort, Elimination*

4. A. Steatorrhea is a clinical finding in the presence celiac disease.
   B. **CORRECT:** Iron deficiency anemia due to blood loss is a clinical finding of PUD.
   C. **CORRECT:** Tarry stools due to intestinal bleeding is a clinical finding of PUD.
   D. **CORRECT:** Epigastric pain described as a gnawing or burning sensation is a clinical manifestation of PUD.
   E. Swollen lymph nodes are a clinical manifestation of many conditions and infections, but not of PUD.

   Ⓝ *NCLEX® Connection: Basic Care and Comfort, Elimination*

5. A. Potatoes are gluten-free and a good choice for a client who has celiac disease.
   B. **CORRECT:** Graham crackers are made from wheat flour. A client who has celiac disease should avoid products that are made from wheat flour.
   C. Wild rice is gluten-free and a good choice for a client who has celiac disease.
   D. Fruits and vegetables without a sauce are gluten-free and are good choices for a client who has celiac disease.

   Ⓝ *NCLEX® Connection: Basic Care and Comfort, Nutrition and Oral Hydration*

Active Learning Scenario Key

Using the ATI Active Learning Template: System Disorder

CLIENT EDUCATION
- The underlying cause of lactose intolerance is an inadequate level of lactase. The enzyme that converts lactose into glucose and galactose is absent or insufficient.
- Manifestations
  ○ Abdominal distension
  ○ Cramps
  ○ Flatus
  ○ Diarrhea
- Foods to limit or avoid include milk, soft cheese, ice cream, cream soups, puddings.

Ⓝ *NCLEX® Connection: Physiological Adaptation, Illness Management*

UNIT 3   ALTERATIONS IN NUTRITION

CHAPTER 14 *Renal Disorders*

Nurses must understand nutritional needs of clients who have renal disorders. It is important to explore dietary needs with the client and recommend modifications related to the disease process. Understanding the role of primary and secondary prevention is essential to successful treatment.

The kidneys have two primary functions: maintaining blood volume and excreting waste products. Other functions include the regulation of acid-base balance, blood pressure, calcium and phosphorous metabolism, and red blood cell production. Kidney damage and/or loss of kidney function have profound effects on the client's nutritional state. Urea is a waste by-product of protein metabolism, and urea levels rise with kidney disease. Monitoring protein intake is critical.

Short-term kidney disease requires nutritional support for healing rather than dietary restrictions. Dietary recommendations are dependent upon the stage of kidney disease.

Nutritional considerations included in this chapter are for chronic kidney disease and end-stage kidney disease, acute kidney injury, nephrotic syndrome, and nephrolithiasis (kidney stones).

Referral to and consultation with a registered dietitian to determine calories, protein, and other nutrients is essential for the client to decrease the risk of malnutrition.

ASSESSMENT/DATA COLLECTION

Chronic kidney disease is distinguished by an increase in blood creatinine. Manifestations include fatigue, back pain, and appetite changes. It is a progressive disorder, characterized by five stages.
- Stage 1: at risk for CKD
- Stage 2: mild CKD
- Stage 3: moderate CKD
- Stage 4: severe CKD
- Stage 5: CKD requiring dialysis or transplant for survival (end-stage kidney disease)

End-stage kidney disease (ESKD) manifestations include fatigue, decreased alertness, anemia, decreased urination, headache, and weight loss.

Acute kidney injury (AKI) manifestations include a decrease in urination, decreased sensation in the extremities, swelling of the lower extremities, and flank pain. It is characterized by rising blood levels of urea and other nitrogenous wastes.

Nephrotic syndrome's most pronounced manifestations are edema and high proteinuria. Other manifestations include hypoalbuminemia, hyperlipidemia, and blood hypercoagulation.

Kidney stones are characterized by sudden, intense pain that is typically located in the flank and is unrelieved by position changes as the stone moves out of the kidney pelvis and down the ureter. Diaphoresis, nausea, and vomiting are common, and there can be blood in the urine. The majority of kidney stones are made of calcium oxalate.

NUTRITIONAL GUIDELINES AND NURSING INTERVENTIONS

General renal considerations

- Monitor kidney parameters for clients who have renal disorders.
  - Nurses should monitor weight daily or as prescribed. Weight is an indicator of fluid status, which is a primary concern. Q EBP
  - Monitor fluid intake, and encourage compliance with fluid restrictions.
  - Nurses should monitor urine output. Placement of an indwelling urinary catheter might be necessary for accurate measurement.
  - Monitor for manifestations of constipation. Fluid restrictions predispose clients to constipation.
- Explain why dietary changes are necessary. Alterations in the intake of protein, calories, sodium, potassium, phosphorus, and other vitamins are required.
- Provide support for the client and family.

Chronic kidney disease (stages 1 to 4)

- Stages 1 to 4 are predialysis and characterized by increasing blood creatinine levels and a decreasing glomerular filtration rate (GFR).

THERAPEUTIC NUTRITION
- Goals of nutritional therapy
  - Slow the progression of CKD.
  - Control blood glucose and hypertension.
  - Help preserve remaining kidney function by limiting the intake of protein, which results in decreased phosphorus levels.
- Restricting phosphorus intake slows the progression of kidney disease. High levels of phosphorus contribute to calcium and phosphorus deposits in the kidneys.
- Protein restriction is essential for clients who have stage 1 to 4 CKD.
  - Slows the progression of kidney disease.
  - Too little protein results in the breakdown of body protein. Carefully determine protein intake.

DIETARY RECOMMENDATIONS

- Restrict sodium intake to maintain blood pressure.
- Restrict potassium intake to prevent hyperkalemia.
- The recommended daily protein intake is 0.8 to 1.0 g/kg/day of ideal body weight.
  - Protein restrictions are decreased as the disease progresses to ESKD, and to decrease the workload on the kidneys.
  - High biologic value proteins are recommended for clients who have CKD to prevent catabolism of muscle tissue. These proteins include eggs, meats, poultry, game, fish, soy, and dairy products.
- Limit meat intake to 5 to 6 oz/day for most males and 4 oz/day for most females.
- Limit dairy products to ½ cup per day.
- Limit high-phosphorus foods (peanut butter, dried peas and beans, bran, cola, chocolate, beer, some whole grains) to one serving or less per day.
- Caution clients to use vitamin and mineral supplements only when recommended by a provider. Avoid high protein sports drinks, energy drinks, or meal supplements. Avoid herbal supplements that can affect bleeding time and blood pressure. Qs

End-stage kidney disease

ESKD, or Stage 5 CKD, occurs when the GFR is less than 15 mL/min and the blood creatinine level steadily rises, and indicates complete kidney failure.

THERAPEUTIC NUTRITION

- The goal of nutritional therapy is to maintain appropriate fluid status, blood pressure, and blood chemistries.
  - A low-protein, low-phosphorus, low-potassium, low-sodium (2 to 3 g/day), fluid-restricted diet is recommended.
  - Consume adequate calories (35 kcal/kg of body weight) to maintain body protein stores.
- Monitor potassium level and replace as needed. Sodium and fluid allowances are determined by blood pressure, weight, blood electrolyte findings, and urine output.
- Achieving a well-balanced diet based on the above guidelines is difficult. The National Renal Diet provides clients with a list of food choices.
- Protein needs increase from 0.6 to 1.0 g/kg before dialysis to 1.2 to 1.5 g/kg, depending on the type of dialysis, once dialysis has begun as protein and amino acids are lost in the dialysate.
  - Fifty percent of protein intake should come from biologic sources (eggs, milk, meat, fish, poultry, soy).
- Restrict phosphorus (700 to 1,200 mg/day).
  - A high protein requirement leads to an increase in phosphorus intake.
  - Foods high in phosphorus are milk products, beef liver, chocolate, nuts, and legumes.
  - Phosphate binders (calcium carbonate, calcium acetate) are taken with all meals and snacks.

- Vitamin D deficiency occurs as the kidneys are unable to convert vitamin D to its active form.
  - This alters the metabolism of calcium, phosphorus, and magnesium, leading to hyperphosphatemia, hypocalcemia, and hypermagnesemia.
  - Calcium supplements will likely be required because foods high in phosphorus (which are restricted) are also high in calcium.

Acute kidney injury

AKI is an abrupt, rapid decline in kidney function caused by trauma, sepsis, poor perfusion, or medications, and usually is reversible. AKI can cause hyponatremia, hyperkalemia, hypocalcemia, and hyperphosphatemia. Fluid overload leading to pulmonary edema is a complication of AKI.

THERAPEUTIC NUTRITION

- Diet therapy for AKI is dependent upon the phase of AKI and its underlying cause. Protein, calories, fluids, potassium, and sodium need to be individualized according to the three phases of AKI (oliguric, diuretic, recovery) and whether the client is receiving dialysis.
- Recommendation is to consume 20 to 30 cal/kg/day of body weight in clients who are in any stage of AKI to maintain energy and demands of stress.
- Simple carbohydrates, fats, oils, and low-protein starches are included in the diet. Provide nonprotein calories in an adequate amount to maintain the client's weight.
- Protein intake can increase to 1 to 1.5 g/kg if the client is receiving dialysis, compared to 0.6 g/kg (40 g/day) for nondialysis clients.
- Potassium and sodium are dependent on urine output, blood values, and if the client is receiving dialysis.
  - Potassium is restricted to 60 to 70 mEq/day when on dialysis.
  - Sodium is restricted to 1 to 2 g/day if not receiving dialysis, and 2 to 4 g/day if receiving dialysis, which also depends on the phase.
  - Calcium requirements are less than 2,000 mg daily if receiving hemodialysis or peritoneal dialysis.
- Fluids are restricted to the client's daily urine output plus 500 mL during the oliguric phase. Fluid needs are increased during the diuretic phase.

Nephrotic syndrome

- Nephrotic syndrome results in the increased excretion of proteins into the urine, resulting in hypoalbuminemia, edema, hyperlipidemia, and blood hypercoagulation. Prolonged protein loss leads to protein malnutrition, anemia, and vitamin D deficiency.
- Diabetes mellitus, kidney damage due to medications or chemicals, autoimmune disorders, and infections can cause nephrotic syndrome.

THERAPEUTIC NUTRITION

- Nutritional therapy goals include minimizing edema, replacing lost nutrients, minimizing kidney damage, controlling hypertension, and preventing protein malnutrition that can lead to muscle catabolism.
- Dietary recommendations indicate sufficient protein and low sodium intake.
  - Adequate amount of protein intake is 0.7 to 1.0 g/kg/day.
  - Soy-based proteins can decrease protein losses and lower blood lipid levels.
  - Low-sodium diet of 2,000 mg/day can help control edema and hypertension.
  - Carbohydrates should provide the majority of the client's daily calories.
  - Cholesterol, trans fat, and saturated fats can be restricted to assist in controlling high lipid levels.
  - Provide a multiple vitamin supplement to replace loss of vitamins with protein excretion. Replace loss of vitamin D with a supplement as needed.

Nephrolithiasis

- The most common type of kidney stone is made of calcium oxalate.
- Contributing factors include inadequate fluid intake, elevated urine pH, and excess excretion through the kidneys of oxalate, calcium, and uric acid.
- Kidney stone formation is more influenced by the amount of oxalate in the client's system than calcium. A client who has an ileostomy has an increased risk of kidney stones.

PREVENTATIVE NUTRITION: Excessive intake of protein, sodium, calcium, and oxalates (rhubarb, spinach, beets) can increase the risk of stone formation.

THERAPEUTIC NUTRITION

- Increasing fluid consumption is the primary intervention for the treatment and prevention of kidney stones. Daily fluid intake should be enough to produce at least 2 L of urine per day. Drink some fluid before bedtime because urine becomes more concentrated at night. This is particularly important for clients who have cystine stones, which requires an even greater daily fluid intake.
- Recommendation for calcium oxalate stone formation is to limit animal protein, excess sodium, alcohol, and caffeine use. Low potassium can contribute to calcium stone formation.
- Foods high in oxalates include spinach, rhubarb, beets, nuts, chocolate, tea, wheat bran, and strawberries, and should be limited in the diet. Avoid megadoses of vitamin C, which increase the amount of oxalate excreted.
- Recommendation for prevention of uric acid stones is to limit foods high in purines, which include lean meats, organ meats, whole grains, and legumes.

Application Exercises

1. A nurse is planning care for a client who has ESKD. Which of the following should the nurse include in the plan of care? (Select all that apply.)
   - A. Monitor the client's weight daily.
   - B. Encourage the client to comply with fluid restrictions.
   - C. Evaluate intake and output.
   - D. Instruct the client on restricting calories from carbohydrates.
   - E. Monitor for constipation.

2. A nurse is teaching a client who has stage 2 chronic kidney disease about dietary management. Which of the following information should the nurse include in the instructions?
   - A. Restrict protein intake.
   - B. Maintain a high-phosphorus diet.
   - C. Increase intake of foods high in potassium.
   - D. Limit dairy products to 1 cup/day.

3. A nurse is teaching a client about protein needs when on dialysis. Which of the following instructions should the nurse include in the teaching? (Select all that apply.)
   - A. Consume 35 kcal/kg of body weight to maintain body protein stores.
   - B. Take phosphate binders when eating protein-rich foods.
   - C. Increase biologic sources of protein (eggs, milk, and soy).
   - D. Increase protein intake by 50% of the recommended dietary allowance (RDA).
   - E. Consume daily protein intake in the morning.

4. A nurse is teaching about diet restrictions to a client who has acute kidney injury and is on hemodialysis. Which of the following recommendations should the nurse include in the teaching?
   - A. Limit calcium intake to 2,500 mg/day.
   - B. Decrease total fat intake to 45% of daily calories.
   - C. Decrease potassium intake to 60 to 70 mEq/kg.
   - D. Limit sodium intake to 4.5 g/day.

5. A nurse is completing discharge teaching about diet and fluid restrictions to a client who has a calcium oxalate-based kidney stone. Which of the following instructions should the nurse include in the teaching?
   - A. Reduce intake of spinach.
   - B. Decrease broccoli intake.
   - C. Increase intake of vitamin C supplements.
   - D. Limit consumption of purine substances.

Active Learning Scenario

A nurse is reviewing teaching for a client who has nephrotic syndrome. What information should the nurse include? Use the ATI Active Learning Template: System Disorder to complete this item.

ALTERATION IN HEALTH (DIAGNOSIS)

COMPLICATIONS: List three.

CLIENT EDUCATION: Include five teaching points.

Application Exercises Key

1. A. **CORRECT:** Monitoring the client's daily weight assists in determining fluid retention.
   B. **CORRECT:** Implementing fluid restriction for a client helps to slow fluid retention.
   C. **CORRECT:** Evaluating I&O helps to determine if there is an increase in fluid retention.
   D. Carbohydrates are not restricted for a client who has ESKD.
   E. **CORRECT:** Constipation often occurs as a result of fluid restrictions.

   Ⓝ NCLEX® Connection: Basic Care and Comfort, Nutrition and Oral Hydration

2. A. **CORRECT:** Restricting protein intake decreases the risk for proteinuria and decreases the workload on the kidney.
   B. A diet high in phosphorus is not recommended because it can contribute to calcium and phosphorus deposits on the kidney.
   C. Eating foods low in potassium is recommended because hyperkalemia occurs with kidney disease.
   D. Dairy products are a protein and sodium source, and are limited to 0.5 cup/day.

   Ⓝ NCLEX® Connection: Basic Care and Comfort, Nutrition and Oral Hydration

3. A. **CORRECT:** To maintain protein stores, the client should consume 35 cal/kg of body weight.
   B. **CORRECT:** Protein consumption increases phosphorus intake. Phosphate binders are recommended with meals.
   C. **CORRECT:** Protein intake should include biologic sources of protein to include eggs, milk, meat, fish, poultry, and soy.
   D. **CORRECT:** The recommended protein intake for a client on dialysis is 50% greater than the RDA because amino acids are lost in the dialysate.
   E. The client should spread protein intake throughout the day to prevent excessive intake of phosphorous and potassium.

   Ⓝ NCLEX® Connection: Basic Care and Comfort, Nutrition and Oral Hydration

4. A. The client receiving hemodialysis should limit calcium intake to less than 2,000 mg/day.
   B. The client should limit total fat intake to 35% of daily calories.
   C. **CORRECT:** The client should limit potassium intake to 60 to 70 mEq/kg.
   D. The client should limit sodium intake to 1 to 4 g/day when receiving dialysis.

   Ⓝ NCLEX® Connection: Basic Care and Comfort, Nutrition and Oral Hydration

5. A. **CORRECT:** The client should reduce intake of foods high in oxalate, such as spinach, which can cause calcium stone formation.
   B. Broccoli is high in calcium but does not cause calcium stone formation and is not restricted in the diet.
   C. Large doses of vitamin C supplements can cause calcium stone formation.
   D. Foods that contain purine, such as organ meats and red wine, cause uric acid stone formation.

   Ⓝ NCLEX® Connection: Health Promotion and Maintenance, Health Promotion/Disease Prevention

Active Learning Scenario Key

Using the ATI Active Learning Template: System Disorder

ALTERATION IN HEALTH (DIAGNOSIS): Nephrotic syndrome is a renal disorder in which there is increased excretion of proteins into the urine.

COMPLICATIONS
- Hypoalbuminemia
- Proteinuria
- Edema
- Hyperlipidemia
- Malnutrition
- Anemia

CLIENT EDUCATION
- Increase protein intake to prevent catabolism of muscle tissue.
- Limit sodium intake to control edema and hypertension.
- Consume foods low in trans fats and cholesterol.
- Consume foods high in carbohydrates to increase calorie intake.
- Take a vitamin supplement to replace vitamin loss that occurs with protein excretion.

Ⓝ NCLEX® Connection: Physiological Adaptation, Illness Management

UNIT 3   ALTERATIONS IN NUTRITION

CHAPTER 15 *Diabetes Mellitus*

Glucose is the body's primary source of energy, and insulin is needed to assist the body in the breakdown of glucose to a form that is used for energy. Diabetes mellitus inhibits the body's production and/or use of insulin. This results in elevated blood glucose levels. Complications of diabetes mellitus are characterized as macrovascular (cardiovascular and cerebrovascular disease) or microvascular (kidney, nerve, and vision problems). For clients who are pregnant, blood glucose control prevents maternal and fetal complications.

The nurse assists the client in identifying lifestyle changes necessary to manage diabetes mellitus, including diet and activity level.

TYPES OF DIABETES MELLITUS

Prediabetes

- Clients who have glucose levels that are elevated above the expected range but below the diagnostic criteria for diabetes mellitus are said to have prediabetes.
- Clients who have prediabetes are encouraged to adopt lifestyle modifications to prevent the development of diabetes mellitus.

Type 1 diabetes mellitus

- Autoimmune disease is triggered by genetic links or a viral infection.
- Damage to or destruction of beta cells of the pancreas results in an absence of insulin production.
- Most often diagnosed before 18 years of age; can occur at any age.

Type 2 diabetes mellitus

- Results from genetic and environmental factors
- Characterized by altered patterns of insulin secretion and decreased cellular uptake of glucose (insulin resistance)

Gestational diabetes mellitus (GDM)

- Glucose intolerance that is recognized during pregnancy, that typically resolves after delivery
- Clients who have a history of GDM have an increased risk for developing diabetes mellitus type 2 later in life.

ASSESSMENT/DATA COLLECTION

Hypoglycemia is a blood glucose level less than 70 mg/dL. It results from taking too much insulin, inadequate food intake, delayed or skipped meals, extra physical activity, or consumption of alcohol without food.
- Manifestations include mild shakiness, mental confusion, sweating, palpitations, headache, lack of coordination, blurred vision, seizures, and coma.

Hyperglycemia is a blood glucose level above the expected reference range. It results from an imbalance with food, medication, and activity, combined with an inadequate amount of insulin production or cells that are insulin-resistant.
- Infection, other illness, and stress can cause an increase in blood glucose.
- Primary manifestations include polydipsia (excessive thirst), polyuria (excessive urination), and polyphagia (excess hunger and eating). As hyperglycemia progresses, ketones (which can be detected in the urine and other manifestations (hyperventilation [Kussmaul respirations], dehydration, fruity odor to the breath, headache, inability to concentrate, decreased levels of consciousness, seizures leading to coma) develop.
- The Somogyi phenomenon is morning hyperglycemia in response to overnight hypoglycemia. Providing a bedtime snack and appropriate insulin dose prevents this phenomenon.
- The dawn phenomenon is an elevation of blood glucose around 0500 to 0600. It results from an overnight release of growth hormone and is treated by increasing the amount of insulin provided during the overnight hours.

Metabolic syndrome is a cluster of factors that increase the risk for diabetes mellitus and cardiovascular complications. Factors include elevated glucose levels, central obesity, hyperlipidemia, hypertension, and low levels of HDL cholesterol. The presence of at least 3 factors indicates metabolic syndrome.

NUTRITIONAL GUIDELINES AND NURSING INTERVENTIONS

Hypoglycemia

- Clients who have hypoglycemia should take 15 to 20 g of a readily absorbable carbohydrate. Qs
  - Two or three glucose tablets (5 g each)
  - Six to ten hard candies
  - ½ cup (4 oz) juice or regular soda
  - 1 tbsp honey or 4 tsp sugar
- Retest the blood glucose in 15 min. If it is less than 70 mg/dL, repeat the above steps. Once levels stabilize, have the client take an additional carbohydrate and protein snack or small meal, depending on the severity of the hypoglycemic episode and whether the next meal is more than 1 hr away.

Hyperglycemia

- Clients who have hyperglycemia should do the following.
  - Notify the provider or go to the emergency department for difficulty concentrating, altered consciousness, or seizure activity.
  - Take medication if forgotten.

GENERAL NUTRITIONAL GUIDELINES

- Coronary heart disease (CHD) is a frequent cause of death among clients who have diabetes. Clients who have diabetes are encouraged to follow a diet that is high in fiber and low in saturated fat, trans fat, and cholesterol to prevent CHD.
- Dietary intake should be individualized according to the client's individual needs, need for weight management, and lipid and glucose patterns. Clients should space food intake throughout the day (regular meals and a snack or snacks). General guidelines follow.
  - **Carbohydrates**
    - Encourage the client to consume carbohydrates found in grains, fruits, legumes, and milk. Limit simple carbohydrates, which include refined grains and sugars.
    - Carbohydrates should be 45% to 65% of total daily caloric intake.
  - **Fats**
    - Clients should eat less saturated and trans fats.
    - Polyunsaturated fatty acids are found in fish. Two or more servings per week are recommended.
    - Consuming foods enriched with plant sterols or stanols can reduce LDL cholesterol.
  - **Fiber**
    - Promote fiber intake (beans, vegetables, oats, whole grains) to improve carbohydrate metabolism and lower cholesterol.
    - Recommendation for fiber intake includes at least 14 g per 1,000 calories.
  - **Protein:** Protein from meats, eggs, fish, nuts, beans, and soy products should comprise 15% to 20% of total caloric intake. Reduce protein intake if needed in clients who have diabetes and kidney failure.
  - **Sodium:** Limit to 2,300 mg/day.
- Encourage clients to eliminate all tobacco use due to the increased risk of cardiovascular disease.
- Moderate alcohol intake can lower the risk for cardiovascular disease. Clients should limit daily alcohol intake to one alcoholic beverage for females or two for males.
  - To avoid hypoglycemia, the client should consume alcohol with a meal or immediately after a meal.
  - Alcoholic beverages should not replace food intake.
- Vitamin and mineral requirements are unchanged for clients who have diabetes. Supplements are recommended for identified deficiencies.

- Artificial sweeteners are acceptable (sucralose, aspartame, saccharin, acesulfame, potassium). Sugar alcohols (xylitol, mannitol, sorbitol) contain some sugar, but not as much as natural sweeteners. Sucrose (table sugar) can be included in a diabetic diet and should be counted in the total calories for the day to ensure antidiabetic medications are sufficient to cover intake.
- Cultural and personal preferences should be considered in planning food intake. Qᴘᴄᴄ
- According to the American Diabetes Association and the Academy of Dietetics and Nutrition, daily nutritional requirements are based on the needs of each client.
- A dietitian works with the client to develop meal planning that meets the client's needs based on healthy food choices. The goal of therapy is to maintain blood glucose levels as close to the expected reference range as possible. Qᴛᴄ
  - The dietitian instructs the client on various dietary methods, including exchange list and carbohydrate counting.
- Using the Food Lists for Diabetes (formerly called Exchange Lists) as a guide for meal planning allows for the incorporation of three basic food groups: protein, carbohydrates, and fats.
  - Each client has a recommended amount of daily exchanges within each group based on the client's needs.

Carbohydrate counting

Carbohydrate counting focuses on counting total grams of carbohydrates in each food item. Many clients find it easier than exchange lists because of the simplicity and flexibility. It does not require the client to learn how much a portion size is.

- One serving equals 15 g of carbohydrates. Clients are free to choose what carbohydrates to consume, but are encouraged to choose a variety of types and include consistent amounts of protein and fats in the diet.
  - Foods that contain 15 g of carbohydrates
    - 1 slice of sandwich bread
    - 1/2 cup cooked pasta
    - 1/2 cup canned fruit in juice (not syrup)
    - 1/4 cup dried fruit
    - 3 cups raw vegetables
    - 1 1/2 cup cooked vegetables
    - 4 to 6 snack crackers
    - 1/2 cup regular ice cream
- With basic carbohydrate counting, a client consumes a specific amount or servings of carbohydrates at each meal and snack.
- With advanced carbohydrate counting, clients calculate mealtime insulin based on the amount of carbohydrates consumed. Clients must be able to perform basic math skills and be willing to check their glucose before each meal to provide a corrective insulin dose, if the glucose level is too high.
- Clients can exchange carbohydrate selections as long as the grams of carbohydrates are the same per serving. Food selections can vary in amount of additional calories from fat and protein each food can contain.

OTHER NURSING INTERVENTIONS

- Provide instructions to the client on the following, and discuss these at subsequent appointments. Q EBP
  - Self-monitoring of blood glucose
  - Dietary and activity recommendations
  - Manifestations and treatment of hypoglycemia and hyperglycemia, to include the importance of taking medications as prescribed
  - Long-term complications of diabetes
  - Psychological implications
  - Community organizations and support groups whose focus is diabetes
- Children who have diabetes require parental support, guidance, and participation. Dietary intake must provide for proper growth and development. Altered nutritional needs during times of growth and fluctuations in eating patterns and activity levels can make management complicated. Q PCC
- For older adult clients, ask questions to determine the presence of deficits that impede adequate nutrition or safe medication administration (cognitive impairment, vision and hearing changes, altered dentition, anorexia, financial barriers).
- For pregnant clients, there must be a balance between maternal blood glucose goals and nutritional needs of pregnancy. Clients might have to monitor blood glucose more often (up to eight times daily).
- Teach proper calibration and use of the self-monitoring of blood glucose, record keeping, and reporting of levels to health care provider.

CLIENT EDUCATION

- Exercise as appropriate and when blood glucose levels are within an acceptable range. Closely monitor blood glucose; decreased medication doses might be required with strenuous exercise to prevent hypoglycemia.
  - Recommendations for adults who have diabetes mellitus includes exercising at least 3 days/week for 150 min total.
  - Adult should not sit for more than 90 min at a time.
- Lose weight if appropriate. It is important for clients who have type 2 diabetes mellitus and have a BMI greater than 25, as it can decrease insulin resistance, improve glucose and lipid levels, and lower blood pressure.
  - Successful weight loss programs include managing calorie intake, exercising, and making lifestyle modifications.
- Be aware of the timing for antidiabetic medications in regard to food intake (before or with meals, or regardless of calorie intake). Take medications at the appropriate time for maximum therapeutic effect.
- Perform self-monitoring of blood glucose. Strict control of glucose can reduce or postpone complications (retinopathy, nephropathy, neuropathy).
- Obtain regular evaluations from the provider.

Application Exercises

1. A nurse is talking with a client who has a new diagnosis of diabetes mellitus type 2 and their caregiver. Which of the following sweeteners should the nurse include as a zero-calorie sweetener option? (Select all that apply.)
   - A. Sucrose
   - B. Aspartame
   - C. Mannitol
   - D. Xylitol
   - E. Sucralose

2. A nurse is assessing a client who is has hypoglycemia. Which of the following findings should the nurse expect?
   - A. Fruity breath odor
   - B. Diaphoresis
   - C. Ketones in urine
   - D. Polyuria

3. A nurse is caring for a client who has diabetes mellitus and reports feeling shaky and weak. The client's blood glucose is 53 mg/dL. Which of the following actions should the nurse take?
   - A. Provide subcutaneous insulin for the client.
   - B. Offer the client 120 mL (4 oz) fruit juice.
   - C. Give the client IV potassium.
   - D. Administer IV sodium bicarbonate.

4. A nurse is reinforcing dietary teaching to a client who has type 2 diabetes mellitus. Which of the following instructions should the nurse include? (Select all that apply.)
   - A. "Carbohydrates should comprise 55% of daily caloric intake."
   - B. "Use hydrogenated oils for cooking."
   - C. "You can add table sugar to cereals."
   - D. "Eat something if you choose to drink alcohol."
   - E. "Use the same portion sizes to exchange carbohydrates."

5. A nurse is teaching a group of clients who have diabetes about meal planning. Which of the following client statements indicates understanding?
   - A. "I will avoid having snacks."
   - B. "I should not eat anything containing sugar."
   - C. "I will not eat fruit canned in syrup."
   - D. "I will not eat more than 2,800 mg of sodium a day."

Active Learning Scenario

A nurse is reviewing the discharge plan for a client who has type 1 diabetes mellitus. How should the nurse use interprofessional care in the plan? Use the ATI Active Learning Template: System Disorder to complete this item.

INTERPROFESSIONAL CARE: Describe the role of another member of the health care team.

CLIENT EDUCATION: Describe three teaching points offered by this member of the health team.

1. A. Common table sugar is sucrose, and it contains about 15 g of carbohydrates per tablespoon.
   B. **CORRECT:** Aspartame is an artificial sweetener that can sweeten foods and beverages without adding calories.
   C. Mannitol is a type of sugar alcohol, which has a low amount of calories (1.6 calories/g).
   D. Xylitol is a type of sugar alcohol, which has a low amount of calories (2.4 calories/g).
   E. **CORRECT:** Sucralose is an artificial sweetener that can sweeten foods and beverages without adding calories.

   Ⓝ *NCLEX® Connection: Physiological Adaptation, Illness Management*

2. A. Fruity breath odor is a manifestation of hyperglycemia.
   B. **CORRECT:** A client who has hypoglycemia can have diaphoresis and cool, clammy skin.
   C. Ketones in the urine is a manifestation of hyperglycemia.
   D. Polyuria (excessive urination) is a manifestation of hyperglycemia.

   Ⓝ *NCLEX® Connection: Reduction of Risk Potential, System Specific Assessments*

3. A. IV insulin is administered for hyperglycemia.
   B. **CORRECT:** The client has manifestations of hypoglycemia. Offer the client 15 to 20 g of carbohydrate, such as 120 mL juice.
   C. IV potassium is administered for hypokalemia.
   D. IV sodium bicarbonate is administered for metabolic acidosis.

   Ⓝ *NCLEX® Connection: Reduction of Risk Potential, System Specific Assessments*

4. A. **CORRECT:** Carbohydrates should be 45% to 65% of total daily calorie intake.
   B. The client should avoid using hydrogenated oils for cooking because they contain trans fatty acids and increase the risk for hyperlipidemia.
   C. **CORRECT:** The client can use table sugar as long as adequate insulin or other agents are provided to cover the sugar intake. The client should count the carbohydrates in the sucrose in the daily carbohydrate count.
   D. **CORRECT:** The client can drink alcohol (one drink/day for females, two drinks/day for males) but should eat something to reduce the risk of hypoglycemia.
   E. **CORRECT:** The client can exchange carbohydrates as long as the total grams of carbohydrates remains the same each day.

   Ⓝ *NCLEX® Connection: Physiological Adaptation, Illness Management*

5. A. Inform the client that a small snack before bedtime might be required to prevent hypoglycemia during the night.
   B. Instruct the client that it is okay to eat some foods containing sugar, but in moderation and included in daily carbohydrate counting.
   C. **CORRECT:** To avoid extra carbohydrate intake, the client should eat fruit that was canned with water or juice rather than syrup, honey, or molasses.
   D. Instruct the client to limit sodium intake to 2,300 mg/day.

   Ⓝ *NCLEX® Connection: Basic Care and Comfort, Nutrition and Oral Hydration*

Using the ATI Active Learning Template: System Disorder

INTERPROFESSIONAL CARE: Dietitian: Development of meal planning based on healthy food choices to meet the client's needs.

CLIENT EDUCATION
- Review of exchange list: Incorporate proteins, carbohydrates, and fats within each group based on the client's needs.
- Review of carbohydrate counting: Consider the total grams of carbohydrates in each food item and the quantity needed for each meal and snack.
- Review information on food labels: Teach how to read food labels to identify amounts of carbohydrates contained in food.

Ⓝ *NCLEX® Connection: Physiological Adaptation, Illness Management*

UNIT 3 ALTERATIONS IN NUTRITION

CHAPTER 16 Cancer and Immunosuppression Disorders

Nurses should be knowledgeable of nutritional needs for clients who have cancer and immunosuppression disorders. Cancer and cancer treatments can affect chewing, swallowing, satiety, digestion, taste, appetite, nutrient absorption, use of glucose, and stool formation (dependent on type).

Protein-calorie malnutrition and body wasting are common secondary diagnoses for clients who have cancer or immunosuppression disorders (HIV/AIDS). Nutritional deficits are a major cause of morbidity and mortality for these clients. Adverse effects of treatments compromise the nutritional status of affected clients. Immunosuppression disorders increase the body's metabolic demands. Alterations in fat storage and metabolism are related to medications used in treatment of the disorder. While subcutaneous fat is lost in the face and extremities, fatty deposits occur in the liver and skeletal muscles.

The goals of nutritional therapy are to minimize the nutritional complications of disease, improve nutritional status, prevent muscle wasting, maintain weight, promote healing, reduce adverse effects, decrease morbidity and mortality, and enhance quality of life and overall effectiveness of treatment therapies. Nutritional plans are individualized for client needs.

ASSESSMENT/DATA COLLECTION

- Current illness and presence of other medical diagnoses
- Nutritional habits, food preferences, and restrictions
- Food allergies
- Height, weight, body mass index (BMI), weight trends

RISK FACTORS

Immunosuppression disorders

- Unprotected sex (HIV)
- Use of contaminated needles (injection substance use [HIV])
- Use of medications that have immunosuppressive effects (cytotoxic medications, corticosteroids, disease modifying immunosuppressive medications)
- History of radiation treatment
- Congenital immune deficiencies

Cancer

- Obesity
- Excessive fat intake
- Sedentary lifestyle
- Consumption of processed meats, red meats, refined grains
- Excessive alcohol intake
- Family history
- History of cigarette smoking

LABORATORY TESTS

Albumin, ferritin, transferrin

NUTRITIONAL GUIDELINES AND NURSING INTERVENTIONS

Immunosuppression

- Monitor the effectiveness of nutrition (weight, BMI, laboratory findings).
- Assist the client to set realistic goals for nutrition and food consumption.
- Instruct the client on strategies to manage adverse effects of treatment.

CLIENT EDUCATION

- Potential food sources of bacteria include raw fruits and vegetables, and undercooked meat, poultry, or eggs. Wash fruits and vegetables. Cook foods thoroughly. Refrigerate perishable foods as soon as possible. Qs
- Make food choices based on nutrition recommendations.

Cancer

Excess body fat stimulates the production of estrogen and progesterone, which can intensify the growth of various cell types and can contribute to breast, gallbladder, colon, prostate, uterine, and kidney cancers.

NURSING ACTIONS: Use semisolid, thickened foods for clients who have dysphagia, and instruct them to sit upright and tilt their head forward when swallowing. Qs

CLIENT EDUCATION
- Eat more on days when feeling better (on "good" days).
- Consume nutritional supplements that are high in protein and/or calories as between-meal snacks. When necessary, use as a meal replacement.
- Increase protein and caloric content of foods.
  ○ Substitute whole milk for water in recipes.
  ○ Add milk, cheese, yogurt, or ice cream to dishes.
  ○ Use peanut butter as a spread for fruits.
  ○ Use yogurt as a topping for fruit.
  ○ Dip meats in eggs, milk, and bread crumbs before cooking.
- **Preventative nutrition**
  ○ Consume adequate dietary fiber (25 to 38 g/day depending on sex and age) to lessen the risk of colon cancer.
  ○ Eliminate tobacco and exposure to loose asbestos to reduce the risk of lung cancer.
  ○ Eat at least 2.5 cups of a variety of fruits and vegetables daily (linked to lowered incidence of many types of cancer and obesity, which affects the risk for cancer development).
    ▪ Foods high in vitamin A (dark green, red, and orange vegetables)
    ▪ Foods high in vitamin C (citrus fruits)
    ▪ Cruciferous vegetables (broccoli, cauliflower, cabbage)
  ○ Consume whole grains rather than processed or refined grains and sugars. Low-fiber foods and foods high in fat can cause a variety of cancers (lung, esophageal, pancreatic, oral cavity, cervical, kidney, bladder, liver, stomach).
  ○ Avoid meat prepared by smoking, pickling, charcoal and grilling, and use of nitrate-containing chemicals (possibly carcinogenic).
  ○ Consume polyunsaturated and monounsaturated fats (found in fish and olive oil), which might be beneficial in lowering the risk of many types of cancer.
  ○ Limit alcohol consumption (associated with many types of cancers).
- **Therapeutic nutrition**
  ○ Cancer can cause anorexia, increased metabolism, and negative nitrogen balance.
  ○ Systemic effects result in poor food intake, increased nutrient and energy needs, and catabolism of body tissues.
  ○ An individualized plan is based on the following. Qpcc
    ▪ Increased caloric needs ranging from 25 to 35 cal/kg (depending on metabolism, activity level, disease state, and ability to absorb nutrients).
    ▪ Protein needs are increased to 1.0 to 2.5 g/kg.
    ▪ Vitamin and mineral supplementation is based upon the client's needs.

HIV/AIDS

The body's response to the inflammatory and immune processes associated with HIV increases nutrient requirements. Malnutrition is common and is one cause of death in clients who have AIDS.
- HIV infection, secondary infection, malignancies, and medication therapies can cause manifestations and adverse effects that impair intake and alter metabolism.
- Decreased nutrient intake occurs due to physical manifestations (anorexia, nausea, vomiting, diarrhea). Psychological manifestations can include depression and dementia.
- Nutritional findings include rapid weight loss, gastrointestinal problems, inadequate intake, increased nutrient needs, food aversions, fad diets, and supplements.
- Poor nutritional status leads to wasting and fever, further increasing susceptibility to secondary infections.
- HIV-associated wasting is characterized by unintended weight loss of 10% and at least one concurrent problem (diarrhea, chronic weakness, or fever) for at least 30 days.
- Diarrhea and malabsorption are prominent concerns in clients who have AIDS.

Therapeutic nutrition
- Creating an individualized plan for the client who has HIV/AIDS is based on reducing unintentional weight loss and wasting.
  ○ Increased caloric needs ranges from 37 to 55 cal/kg.
  ○ A high-protein diet is recommended with amounts varying from 1.2 to 2.0 g/kg/day.
  ○ Intake of a multivitamin that meets 100% of the recommended daily servings is sufficient, unless a specific deficiency is identified.
- Enteral feedings are used if the client is unable to consume sufficient nutrients, calories, and fluid.
- Liberal fluid intake is extremely important to prevent dehydration.

CLIENT EDUCATION: Consume small, frequent meals that are composed of high-protein, high-calorie, nutrient-dense foods.

COMPLICATIONS

Early satiety and anorexia

CLIENT EDUCATION
- Eat small amounts of high-protein foods loaded with calories and nutrients.
- Try to consume food in the morning when appetite is best.
- Avoid food odors.
- Do not fill up on low-calorie foods (liquids, broth, high-roughage foods containing water).
- Eat cool or room temperature foods.

Mouth ulcers and stomatitis

CLIENT EDUCATION
- Use a soft toothbrush to clean teeth after eating and at bedtime.
- Avoid mouth washes that contain alcohol.
- Omit acidic, spicy, dry, or coarse foods.
- Include cold or room-temperature foods in the diet.
- Cut food into small bites.
- Try using straws.
- Replace meals with high-calorie/protein drinks.
- Use well-fitting dentures.
- Prepare foods that are cooked until tender and soft.
- Add gravies, broth, and a variety of mild sauces to moistened prepared foods.

Fatigue

CLIENT EDUCATION
- Eat a large, calorie-dense breakfast when energy level is the highest.
- Conserve energy by eating foods that are easy to prepare.
- Use a meal delivery service.

Food aversions

CLIENT EDUCATION: Eat foods that are well-tolerated and liked prior to treatments (chemotherapy, radiation). Qpcc

Taste alterations and thick saliva

CLIENT EDUCATION
- Try adding foods that are tart (citrus juices).
- Eat small, frequent meals.
- Try using sauces and seasonings for added flavor.
- Use plastic utensils for eating.
- Suck on mints, candy, or chew gum to remove bad taste in mouth.
- Sweeten meat with apple or cranberry sauce.

Nausea, vomiting

CLIENT EDUCATION
- Eat cold or room-temperature foods.
- Try high-carbohydrate, low-fat foods.
- Avoid fried foods.
- Do not eat prior to chemotherapy or radiation.
- Take prescribed antiemetic medication.
- Sit up for 1 hr after a meal.
- Sip on fluids throughout the day. Try ginger ale or ginger tea.

Diarrhea

CLIENT EDUCATION
- Ensure adequate intake of liquids throughout the day to replace losses.
- Avoid foods that can exacerbate diarrhea (foods high in roughage).
- Consume foods high in pectin to increase the bulk of the stool and to lengthen transition time in the colon.
- Limit caffeine, hot or cold drinks, and fatty foods.

Application Exercises

1. A nurse is teaching a client who has cancer about ways to increase protein and calories in foods. Which of the following actions should the nurse include? (Select all that apply.)

   A. Use peanut butter as a spread on crackers.

   B. Add water in place of milk in soups.

   C. Top fruit with yogurt.

   D. Dip chicken in eggs before cooking.

   E. Sprinkle cheese on a baked potato.

2. A nurse is teaching a community program on nutritional guidelines for cancer prevention. Which of the following instructions should the nurse include? (Select all that apply.)

   A. Eat foods high in vitamin A.

   B. Add cruciferous vegetables.

   C. Increase intake of red meats

   D. Use oil high in saturated fat.

   E. Consume refined grains.

3. A nurse in an oncology clinic is caring for a client who is undergoing treatment for cancer and reports difficulty eating due to inability to taste food. Which of the following interventions should the nurse recommend?

   A. Avoid citrus juices.

   B. Use plastic utensils to eat.

   C. Eat foods that are warm.

   D. Increase foods high in pectin.

4. A nurse is teaching a client who is undergoing cancer treatment about interventions to manage stomatitis. Which of the following statements by the client indicates understanding of the teaching?

   A. "I will try chewing larger pieces of food."

   B. "I will avoid toasting my bread."

   C. "I will consume more food in the morning."

   D. "I will add more citrus foods to my diet."

5. A nurse is collecting data from a client who has suspected HIV-associated muscle wasting. Which of the following findings supports this diagnosis?

   A. BMI 26

   B. Fecal impaction

   C. Report of fever for 30 days

   D. Report of high alcohol consumption

Active Learning Scenario

A nurse in an oncology clinic is reviewing dietary management with a group of clients who have cancer and are undergoing treatment. What instructions should the nurse include in this discussion? Use the ATI Active Learning Template: System Disorder to complete this item.

CLIENT EDUCATION

• Describe three effects of cancer on nutrition.

• Describe three nutritional needs.

• Describe three activities that promote improved nutrition.

Application Exercises Key

1. A. **CORRECT:** Peanut butter adds calories and protein to fruit slices or crackers.
    B. The client should substitute whole milk, cream, and/or hard-boiled eggs to soups and sauces to increase protein and calories.
    C. **CORRECT:** Yogurt adds protein and calories to fruit.
    D. **CORRECT:** Eggs add protein and calories to chicken, fish, or meat.
    E. **CORRECT:** Cheese adds protein and calories to vegetables.

    Ⓝ *NCLEX® Connection: Basic Care and Comfort, Nutrition and Oral Hydration*

2. A. **CORRECT:** Consuming foods high in vitamin A (apricots, carrots, leafy green vegetables) reduces the risk of cancer.
    B. **CORRECT:** Consuming cruciferous vegetables, such as broccoli and cabbage, reduces the risk the risk of cancer.
    C. Increased consumption of red meat can increase the risk for cancer.
    D. The use of polyunsaturated and monounsaturated fats is beneficial in lowering the risk of many types of cancer, while foods high in saturated fats are associated with an increased risk of cancer.
    E. Consuming whole grains reduces the risk for colon cancer.

    Ⓝ *NCLEX® Connection: Health Promotion and Maintenance, Health Promotion/Disease Prevention*

3. A. Add tart foods, such as citrus, to the diet to increase food taste and reduce the occurrence of a metallic taste.
    B. **CORRECT:** The use of plastic utensils when eating can enhance taste sensations for the client undergoing cancer treatment and reduce the occurrence of a metallic taste.
    C. Eating cold or room-temperature foods improves taste sensation.
    D. Add pectin-rich foods to increase bulk of the stool and lengthen transition time in the colon.

    Ⓝ *NCLEX® Connection: Basic Care and Comfort, Nutrition and Oral Hydration*

4. A. The client should be encouraged to cut food into small pieces to reduce irritation to mucous membranes.
    B. **CORRECT:** Dry, coarse foods such as toast can worsen the manifestations of stomatitis.
    C. This intervention is indicated for the client who has fatigue due to cancer treatment.
    D. Acidic or spicy foods irritate the mucous membranes of the client who has stomatitis due to cancer treatment.

    Ⓝ *NCLEX® Connection: Basic Care and Comfort, Nutrition and Oral Hydration*

5. A. A BMI of 26 is within the expected reference range; a weight loss of at least 10% is one factor required to diagnose HIV-associated muscle wasting.
    B. Diarrhea is common for a client who has HIV-associated muscle wasting.
    C. **CORRECT:** Report of fever or other condition for 30 days, in addition to a specific weight loss, indicates HIV-associated muscle wasting.
    D. Alcohol consumption is not a factor used to diagnose HIV-associated muscle wasting.

    Ⓝ *NCLEX® Connection: Physiological Adaptation, Alterations in Body Systems*

Active Learning Scenario Key

Using the ATI Active Learning Template: System Disorder

CLIENT EDUCATION

Effects of cancer on nutrition
- Causes anorexia
- Increases metabolism
- Causes negative nitrogen balance

Nutritional needs
- Increased calories (25 to 35 cal/kg)
- Increased protein (1 to 2.5 g/kg)
- Vitamin and mineral supplementation

Activities
- Eat more on days when feeling better.
- Consume nutritional supplements that are high in protein and/or calories between meals and/or use as meal replacement.
- Substitute whole milk for water in recipes.
- Add milk, cheese, yogurt, or ice cream to foods when cooking.
- Add peanut butter and yogurt as a spread/topping on fruits.
- Coat meats in eggs, milk, and bread crumbs before cooking.
- Treat cancer-associated complications (early satiety, anorexia, mouth ulcers, stomatitis, fatigue, food aversions, altered taste, thick saliva, nausea, vomiting, diarrhea).

Ⓝ *NCLEX® Connection: Physiological Adaptation, Illness Management*

References

Berman, A., Snyder, S., & Frandsen, G. (2016). *Kozier & Erb's fundamentals of nursing: Concepts, process, and practice* (10th ed.). Upper Saddle River, NJ: Prentice-Hall.

Burchum, J. R., & Rosenthal, L. D. (2019). *Lehne's pharmacology for nursing care* (10th ed.). St. Louis, MO.

Dudek, S. G. (2018). *Nutrition essentials for nursing practice* (8th ed.). Philadelphia: Wolters Kluwer.

Grodner, M., Escott-Stump, S., & Dorner, S. (2016). *Nutritional foundations and clinical applications of nutrition: A nursing approach* (6th ed.). St. Louis, MO: Mosby

Hinkle, J. L., & Cheever, K. H. (2018). *Brunner and Suddarth's textbook of medical-surgical nursing* (14th ed.). Philadelphia: Wolters Kluwer.

Hockenberry, M. J., & Wilson, D. (2015). *Wong's nursing care of infants and children* (10th ed.). St. Louis, MO: Mosby.

Ignatavicius, D. D., Workman, M.L., & Rebar, C. R. (2018). Medical-Surgical nursing: Concepts for Interprofessional collaborative care. (9th Ed). St. Louis, MO.

Pagana, K. D., & Pagana, T. J. (2018). *Mosby's manual of diagnostic and laboratory tests* (6th ed.). St. Louis, MO: Elsevier.

Potter, P. A., Perry, A. G., Stockert, P., & Hall, A. (2017). *Fundamentals of nursing* (9th ed.). St. Louis, MO: Elsevier.

Touhy, T. A., & Jett, K. F. (2016). *Ebersole & Hess' toward healthy aging: Human needs and nursing response* (9th ed.). St. Louis, MO: Elsevier.

United States Department of Agriculture (USDA). (2013). Sausages and food safety. Retrieved from https://www.fsis.usda.gov/wps/wcm/connect/fsis-content/internet/main/topics/food-safety-education/get-answers/food-safety-fact-sheets/meat-preparation/sausages-and-food-safety/ct_index

U. S. Food and Drug administration. (2016). Food labeling: Revision of the nutrition and supplement facts labels. https://www.regulations.gov/document?D=FDA-2012-N-1210-0875

U. S. Food and Drug administration. (2018). Refrigerator & freezer storage chart. Retrieved from https://www.fda.gov/downloads/food/foodborneillnesscontaminants/ucm109315.pdf

U. S. Food and Drug administration. (2017). Surplus, salvaged, and donated foods: Safety tips. Retrieved from https://www.fda.gov/Food/ResourcesForYou/Consumers/ucm197835.htm

U. S. Food and Drug administration. (2017). Safe food handling: What you need to know. Retrieved from https://www.fda.gov/downloads/Food/FoodborneIllnessContaminants/BuyStoreServeSafeFood/UCM440123.pdf

U. S. Food and Drug administration. (2018). Produce: selecting and serving it safely. Retrieved from https://www.fda.gov/food/foodborneillnesscontaminants/buystoreservesafefood/ucm114299.htm

STUDENT NAME _____

CONCEPT_____ REVIEW MODULE CHAPTER_____

Related Content
(E.G., DELEGATION, LEVELS OF PREVENTION, ADVANCE DIRECTIVES)

Underlying Principles

Nursing Interventions
WHO? WHEN? WHY? HOW?

STUDENT NAME _____

PROCEDURE NAME _____ REVIEW MODULE CHAPTER_____

Description of Procedure

Indications

CONSIDERATIONS

Nursing Interventions (pre, intra, post)

Interpretation of Findings

Client Education

Potential Complications

Nursing Interventions

STUDENT NAME _____

DEVELOPMENTAL STAGE _____ REVIEW MODULE CHAPTER_____

EXPECTED GROWTH AND DEVELOPMENT

Physical Development	Cognitive Development	Psychosocial Development	Age-Appropriate Activities

Health Promotion

Immunizations	Health Screening	Nutrition	Injury Prevention

STUDENT NAME _____

MEDICATION _____ REVIEW MODULE CHAPTER_____

CATEGORY CLASS_____

PURPOSE OF MEDICATION

Expected Pharmacological Action

Therapeutic Use

Complications

Medication Administration

Contraindications/Precautions

Nursing Interventions

Interactions

Client Education

Evaluation of Medication Effectiveness

STUDENT NAME _____

SKILL NAME_____ REVIEW MODULE CHAPTER_____

Description of Skill

Indications

CONSIDERATIONS

Nursing Interventions (pre, intra, post)

Outcomes/Evaluation

Client Education

Potential Complications

Nursing Interventions

STUDENT NAME _____

DISORDER/DISEASE PROCESS _____ REVIEW MODULE CHAPTER_____

Alterations in Health (Diagnosis)	Pathophysiology Related to Client Problem	Health Promotion and Disease Prevention

ASSESSMENT

Risk Factors

Expected Findings

Laboratory Tests

Diagnostic Procedures

SAFETY CONSIDERATIONS

PATIENT-CENTERED CARE

Nursing Care

Medications

Client Education

Therapeutic Procedures

Interprofessional Care

Complications

ACTIVE LEARNING TEMPLATE: *Therapeutic Procedure*

STUDENT NAME _____

PROCEDURE NAME _____ REVIEW MODULE CHAPTER_____

Description of Procedure

Indications

CONSIDERATIONS

Nursing Interventions (pre, intra, post)

Outcomes/Evaluation

Client Education

Potential Complications

Nursing Interventions

Concept Analysis

STUDENT NAME _____

CONCEPT ANALYSIS_____

Defining Characteristics

Antecedents

(WHAT MUST OCCUR/BE IN PLACE FOR
CONCEPT TO EXIST/FUNCTION PROPERLY)

Negative Consequences

(RESULTS FROM IMPAIRED ANTECEDENT —
COMPLETE WITH FACULTY ASSISTANCE)

Related Concepts

(REVIEW LIST OF CONCEPTS AND IDENTIFY, WHICH
CAN BE AFFECTED BY THE STATUS OF THIS CONCEPT
— COMPLETE WITH FACULTY ASSISTANCE)

Exemplars

Nursing Leadership and Management
REVIEW MODULE EDITION 8.0

Contributors

Honey C. Holman, MSN, RN

Debborah Williams, MSN, RN

Sheryl Sommer, PhD, RN, CNE

Janean Johnson, MSN, RN, CNE

Brenda S. Ball, MEd, BSN, RN

Terri Lemon, DNP, MSN, RN

Consultants

Tracey Bousquet, BSN, RN

Julie Traynor, MSN, RN

REPRINTED APRIL 2021

Director of content review: Kristen Lawler

Director of development: Derek Prater

Project management: Tiffany Pavlik, Shannon Tierney

Coordination of content review: Honey C. Holman, Debborah Williams

Copy editing: Kelly Von Lunen, Bethany Phillips, Kya Rodgers

Layout: Spring Lenox, Maureen Bradshaw, Bethany Phillips

Illustrations: Randi Hardy

Online media: Brant Stacy, Ron Hanson, Britney Fuller, Barry Wilson

Cover design: Jason Buck

Interior book design: Spring Lenox

IMPORTANT NOTICE TO THE READER

User's Guide

Welcome to the Assessment Technologies Institute® Nursing Leadership and Management Review Module Edition 8.0. The mission of ATI's Content Mastery Series® Review Modules is to provide user-friendly compendiums of nursing knowledge that will:
- Help you locate important information quickly.
- Assist in your learning efforts.
- Provide exercises for applying your nursing knowledge.
- Facilitate your entry into the nursing profession as a newly licensed nurse.

This newest edition of the Review Modules has been redesigned to optimize your learning experience. We've fit more content into less space and have done so in a way that will make it even easier for you to find and understand the information you need.

ORGANIZATION

Chapters in this Review Module use a nursing concepts organizing framework, beginning with an overview describing the central concept and its relevance to nursing. Subordinate themes are covered in outline form to demonstrate relationships and present the information in a clear, succinct manner. Some chapters have sections that group related concepts and contain their own overviews. These sections are included in the table of contents.

ACTIVE LEARNING SCENARIOS AND APPLICATION EXERCISES

Each chapter includes opportunities for you to test your knowledge and to practice applying that knowledge. Active Learning Scenario exercises pose a nursing scenario and then direct you to use an ATI Active Learning Template (included at the back of this book) to record the important knowledge a nurse should apply to the scenario. An example is then provided to which you can compare your completed Active Learning Template. The Application Exercises include NCLEX-style questions (multiple-choice and multiple-select items), providing you with opportunities to practice answering the kinds of questions you might expect to see on ATI assessments or the NCLEX. After the Application Exercises, an answer key is provided, along with rationales.

NCLEX® CONNECTIONS

To prepare for the NCLEX, it is important to understand how the content in this Review Module is connected to the NCLEX test plan. You can find information on the detailed test plan at the National Council of State Boards of Nursing's website, www.ncsbn.org. When reviewing content in this Review Module, regularly ask yourself, "How does this content fit into the test plan, and what types of questions related to this content should I expect?"

To help you in this process, we've included NCLEX Connections at the beginning of each unit and with each question in the Application Exercises Answer Keys. The NCLEX Connections at the beginning of each unit point out areas of the detailed test plan that relate to the content within that unit. The NCLEX Connections attached to the Application Exercises Answer Keys demonstrate how each exercise fits within the detailed content outline.

These NCLEX Connections will help you understand how the detailed content outline is organized, starting with major client needs categories and subcategories and followed by related content areas and tasks. The major client needs categories are:
- Safe and Effective Care Environment
  - Management of Care
  - Safety and Infection Control
- Health Promotion and Maintenance
- Psychosocial Integrity
- Physiological Integrity
  - Basic Care and Comfort
  - Pharmacological and Parenteral Therapies
  - Reduction of Risk Potential
  - Physiological Adaptation

An NCLEX Connection might, for example, alert you that content within a chapter is related to:
- Management of Care
  - Advance Directives
    - Provide clients with information about advance directives.

QSEN COMPETENCIES

As you use the Review Modules, you will note the integration of the Quality and Safety Education for Nurses (QSEN) competencies throughout the chapters. These competencies are integral components of the curriculum of many nursing programs in the United States and prepare you to provide safe, high-quality care as a newly licensed nurse. Icons appear to draw your attention to the six QSEN competencies.

Safety: The minimization of risk factors that could cause injury or harm while promoting quality care and maintaining a secure environment for clients, self, and others.

Patient-Centered Care: The provision of caring and compassionate, culturally sensitive care that addresses clients' physiological, psychological, sociological, spiritual, and cultural needs, preferences, and values.

Evidence-Based Practice: The use of current knowledge from research and other credible sources, on which to base clinical judgment and client care.

Informatics: The use of information technology as a communication and information-gathering tool that supports clinical decision-making and scientifically based nursing practice.

Quality Improvement: Care related and organizational processes that involve the development and implementation of a plan to improve health care services and better meet clients' needs.

Teamwork and Collaboration: The delivery of client care in partnership with multidisciplinary members of the health care team to achieve continuity of care and positive client outcomes.

ICONS

Icons are used throughout the Review Module to draw your attention to particular areas. Keep an eye out for these icons.

(N) This icon is used for NCLEX Connections.

(G) This icon indicates gerontological considerations, or knowledge specific to the care of older adult clients.

Qs This icon is used for content related to safety and is a QSEN competency. When you see this icon, take note of safety concerns or steps that nurses can take to ensure client safety and a safe environment.

Qpcc This icon is a QSEN competency that indicates the importance of a holistic approach to providing care.

Qebp This icon, a QSEN competency, points out the integration of research into clinical practice.

Qi This icon is a QSEN competency and highlights the use of information technology to support nursing practice.

Qqi This icon is used to focus on the QSEN competency of integrating planning processes to meet clients' needs.

Qtc This icon highlights the QSEN competency of care delivery using an interprofessional approach.

M◇ This icon appears at the top-right of pages and indicates availability of an online media supplement (a graphic, animation, or video). If you have an electronic copy of the Review Module, this icon will appear alongside clickable links to media supplements. If you have a hard copy version of the Review Module, visit www.atitesting.com for details on how to access these features.

FEEDBACK

ATI welcomes feedback regarding this Review Module. Please provide comments to comments@atitesting.com.

As needed updates to the Review Modules are identified, changes to the text are made for subsequent printings of the book and for subsequent releases of the electronic version. For the printed books, print runs are based on when existing stock is depleted. For the electronic versions, a number of factors influence the update schedule. As such, ATI encourages faculty and students to refer to the Review Module addendums for information on what updates have been made. These addendums, which are available in the Help/FAQs on the student site and the Resources/eBooks & Active Learning on the faculty site, are updated regularly and always include the most current information on updates to the Review Modules.

Table of Contents

When reviewing the following chapter, keep in mind the relevant topics and tasks of the NCLEX outline, in particular:

Management of Care

ASSIGNMENT, DELEGATION AND SUPERVISION

Evaluate delegated tasks to ensure correct completion of activity.

Evaluate effectiveness of staff members' time management skills.

CASE MANAGEMENT: Practice and advocate for cost effective care.

CONCEPTS OF MANAGEMENT

Manage conflict among clients and health care staff.

Identify roles/responsibilities of health care team members.

ESTABLISHING PRIORITIES

Apply knowledge of pathophysiology when establishing priorities for interventions with multiple clients.

Prioritize the delivery of client care.

PERFORMANCE IMPROVEMENT (QUALITY IMPROVEMENT): Participate in performance improvement projects and quality improvement processes.

CHAPTER 1 # Managing Client Care

Managing client care requires leadership, management skills, and knowledge to effectively coordinate and carry out client care.

To effectively manage client care, a nurse must develop knowledge and skills in several areas, including leadership, management, critical thinking, clinical reasoning, clinical judgment, prioritization, time management, assigning, delegating, supervising, staff education, quality improvement, performance appraisal, peer review, disciplinary action, conflict resolution, and cost-effective care.

Leadership and management

- Management is the process of planning, organizing, directing, and coordinating the work within an organization.
- Leadership is the ability to inspire others to achieve a desired outcome.
- Effective managers usually possess good leadership skills. However, effective leaders are not always in a management position.
- Managers have formal positions of power and authority. Leaders might have only the informal power afforded them by their peers.
- One cannot be a leader without followers.

LEADERSHIP

LEADERSHIP STYLES

Most can be categorized as autocratic/authoritarian, democratic, or laissez-faire. The nurse might need to use any of these leadership styles depending on the situation.

Autocratic/authoritarian

- Makes decisions for the group.
- Motivates by coercion.
- Communication occurs down the chain of command, or from the highest management level downward through other managers to employees.
- Work output by staff is usually high: good for crisis situations and bureaucratic settings.
- Effective for employees with little or no formal education.

Democratic

- Includes the group when decisions are made. Qᴛᴄ
- Motivates by supporting staff achievements.
- Communication occurs up and down the chain of command.
- Work output by staff is usually of good quality when cooperation and collaboration are necessary.

Laissez-faire

- Makes very few decisions, and does little planning.
- Motivation is largely the responsibility of individual staff members.
- Communication occurs up and down the chain of command and between group members.
- Work output is low unless an informal leader evolves from the group.
- Effective with professional employees.

CHARACTERISTICS OF LEADERS

- Initiative
- Inspiration
- Energy
- Positive attitude
- Communication skills
- Respect
- Problem-solving and critical-thinking skills
- A combination of personality traits and leadership skills
- Leaders influence willing followers to move toward a goal.
- Leaders have goals that might differ from those of the organization.
- **Transformational leaders** empower and inspire followers to achieve a common, long-term vision.
- **Transactional leaders** focus on immediate problems, maintaining the status quo and using rewards to motivate followers.
- **Authentic leaders** inspire others to follow them by modeling a strong internal moral code.

Emotional intelligence

- Emotional intelligence is the ability of an individual to perceive and manage the emotions of self and others.
- The nurse must be able to perceive and understand their own emotions and the emotions of the client and family in order to provide client-centered care. Qᴘᴄᴄ
- Emotional intelligence is also an important characteristic of the successful nurse leader.
- Emotional intelligence is developed through understanding the concept and applying it to practice in everyday situations.

The emotionally intelligent leader:
- Has insight into the emotions of members of the team.
- Understands the perspective of others.
- Encourages constructive criticism and is open to new ideas.
- Manages emotions and channels them in a positive direction, which in turn helps the team accomplish its goals.
- Is committed to the delivery of high-quality client care.
- Refrains from judgment in controversial or emotionally-charged situations until facts are gathered.

MANAGEMENT

The five major management functions are planning, organizing, staffing, directing, and controlling.

PLANNING: The decisions regarding what needs to be done, how it will be done, and who is going to do it

ORGANIZING: The organizational structure that determines the lines of authority, channels of communication, and where decisions are made

STAFFING: The acquisition and management of adequate staff and staffing mix

DIRECTING: The leadership role assumed by a manager that influences and motivates staff to perform assigned roles

CONTROLLING: The evaluation of staff performance and evaluation of unit goals to ensure identified outcomes are being met

CHARACTERISTICS OF MANAGERS

- Hold formal positions of authority and power
- Possess clinical expertise
- Network with members of the team
- Coach subordinates
- Make decisions about the function of the organization, including resources, budget, hiring, and firing

Critical thinking

Critical thinking is used when analyzing client issues and problems. Thinking skills include interpretation, analysis, evaluation, inference, and explanation. These skills assist the nurse to determine the most appropriate action to take.

- Critical thinking reflects upon the meaning of statements, examines available data, and uses reason to make informed decisions.
- Critical thinking is necessary to reflect and evaluate from a broader scope of view.
- Sometimes one must think "outside the box" to find solutions that are best for clients, staff, and the organization.

Clinical reasoning

- Clinical reasoning is the mental process used when analyzing the elements of a clinical situation and using analysis to make a decision. The nurse continues to use clinical reasoning to make decisions as the client's situation changes.
- Clinical reasoning supports the clinical decision-making process by:
  ○ Guiding the nurse through the process of assessing and compiling data.
  ○ Selecting and discarding data based on relevance.
  ○ Using nursing knowledge to make decisions about client care. Problem solving is a part of decision-making.

Clinical judgment

- Clinical judgment is the decision made regarding a course of action based on a critical analysis of data.
- Clinical judgment considers the client's needs when deciding to take an action, or modify an intervention based on the client's response.
- The nurse uses clinical judgment to:
  ○ Analyze data and related evidence.
  ○ Ascertain the meaning of the data and evidence.
  ○ Apply knowledge to a clinical situation.
  ○ Determine client outcomes desired and/or achieved as indicated by evidence-based practices. Qᴇʙᴘ

PRIORITIZATION AND TIME MANAGEMENT

- Nurses must continuously set and reset priorities in order to meet the needs of multiple clients and to maintain client safety. Qs
- Priority setting requires that decisions be made regarding the order in which:
  ○ Clients are seen.
  ○ Assessments are completed.
  ○ Interventions are provided.
  ○ Steps in a client procedure are completed.
  ○ Components of client care are completed.
- Establishing priorities in nursing practice requires that the nurse make these decisions based on evidence obtained:
  ○ During shift reports and other communications with members of the health care team.
  ○ Through careful review of documents.
  ○ By continuously and accurately collecting client data.

PRIORITIZATION PRINCIPLES IN CLIENT CARE

Prioritize systemic before local ("life before limb").

Prioritizing interventions for a client in shock over interventions for a client who has a localized limb injury

Prioritize acute (less opportunity for physical adaptation) before chronic (greater opportunity for physical adaptation).

Prioritizing the care of a client who has a new injury/illness (mental confusion, chest pain) or an acute exacerbation of a previous illness over the care of a client who has a long-term chronic illness

Prioritize actual problems before potential future problems.

Prioritizing administration of medication to a client experiencing acute pain over ambulation of a client at risk for thrombophlebitis

Listen carefully to clients and don't assume.

Asking a client who has a new diagnosis of diabetes mellitus what they feel is most important to learn about disease management.

Recognize and respond to trends vs. transient findings.

> Recognizing a gradual deterioration in a client's level of consciousness and/or Glasgow Coma Scale score

Recognize indications of medical emergencies and complications vs. expected findings.

> Recognizing indications of increasing intracranial pressure in a client who has a new diagnosis of a stroke vs. the findings expected following a stroke

Apply clinical knowledge to procedural standards to determine the priority action.

> Recognizing that the timing of administration of antidiabetic and antimicrobial medications is more important than administration of some other medications

PRIORITY-SETTING FRAMEWORKS

Maslow's hierarchy (1.1) ○PCC

The nurse should consider this hierarchy of human needs when prioritizing interventions. For example, the nurse should prioritize a client's:
- Need for airway, oxygenation (or breathing), circulation, and potential for disability over need for shelter.
- Need for a safe and secure environment over a need for socialization.

Airway breathing circulation (ABC) framework

- The ABC framework identifies, in order, the three basic needs for sustaining life.
  ○ An open airway is necessary for breathing, so it is the highest priority.
  ○ Breathing is necessary for oxygenation of the blood to occur.
  ○ Circulation is necessary for oxygenated blood to reach the body's tissues.
- The severity of manifestations should also be considered when determining priorities. A severe circulation problem can take priority over a minor breathing problem.
- Some frameworks also include a "D" for disability and "E" for exposure.

PRIORITY INTERVENTIONS
- **First: Airway**
  ○ Identify an airway concern (obstruction, stridor).
  ○ Establish a patent airway if indicated.
  ○ Recognize that 3 to 5 min without oxygen causes irreversible brain damage secondary to cerebral anoxia.
- **Second: Breathing**
  ○ Assess the effectiveness of breathing (apnea, depressed respiratory rate).
  ○ Intervene as needed (reposition, administer naloxone).
- **Third: Circulation**
  ○ Identify circulation concern (hypotension, dysrhythmia, inadequate cardiac output, compartment syndrome).
  ○ Institute actions to reverse or minimize circulatory alteration.

- **Fourth: Disability**
  ○ Assess for current or evolving disability (neurological deficits, stroke in evolution).
  ○ Implement actions to slow down development of disability.
- **Fifth: Exposure**
  ○ Remove the client's clothing to allow for a complete assessment or resuscitation.
  ○ Implement measures to reduce the risk for hypothermia (provide warm blankets and IV solutions or use cooling measures for clients exposed to extreme heat).

Safety/risk reduction ○s

- Look first for a safety risk. For example, is there a finding that suggests a risk for airway obstruction, hypoxia, bleeding, infection, or injury?
- Next ask, "What's the risk to the client?" and "How significant is the risk compared to other posed risks?"
- Give priority to responding to whatever finding poses the greatest (or most imminent) risk to the client's physical well-being.

Assessment/data collection first

Use the nursing process to gather pertinent information prior to making a decision regarding a plan of action. For example, determine if additional information is needed prior to calling the provider to ask for pain medication for a client.

Survival potential

- Use this framework for situations in which health resources are extremely limited (mass casualty, disaster triage).
- Give priority to clients who have a reasonable chance of survival with prompt intervention. Clients who have a limited likelihood of survival even with intense intervention are assigned the lowest priority.

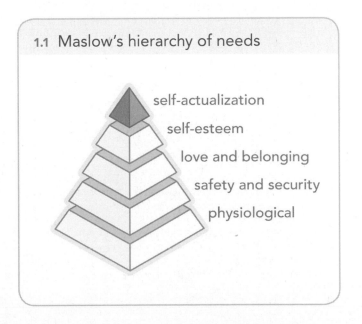

1.1 Maslow's hierarchy of needs

self-actualization
self-esteem
love and belonging
safety and security
physiological

Least restrictive/least invasive

- Select interventions that maintain client safety while posing the least amount of restriction to the client. For example, if a client who has a high fall risk index is getting out of bed without assistance, move the client closer to the nurses' work area rather than choosing to apply restraints.
- Select interventions that are the least invasive. For example, bladder training for the incontinent client is a better option than an indwelling urinary catheter.

Acute vs. chronic, urgent vs. nonurgent, stable vs. unstable

- A client who has an acute problem takes priority over a client who has a chronic problem.
- A client who has an urgent need takes priority over a client who has a nonurgent need.
- A client who has unstable findings takes priority over a client who has stable findings.

Evidence-based practice

- Use current data to make informed clinical decisions to provide the best practice. Best practice is determined by current research collected from several sources that have desirable outcomes.
- Use knowledge of evidence-based practice to guide prioritization of care and interventions (responding to clients experiencing wound dehiscence or crisis). For example, initiating CPR in the proper steps for a client experiencing cardiac arrest.

Methods to promote evidence-based practice
- Use a variety of sources of research.
- Keep current on new research by reading professional journals and collaborating with other nurses and professionals in other disciplines.
- Change traditional nursing practice with new research-based practices.

TIME MANAGEMENT

Organize care according to client care needs and priorities. QPCC
- What must be done immediately (administration of analgesic or antiemetic, assessment of unstable client)?
- What must be done by a specific time to ensure client safety, quality care, and compliance with facility policies and procedures (routine medication administration, vital signs, blood glucose monitoring)?
- What must be done by the end of the shift (ambulation of the client, discharge and/or discharge teaching, dressing change)?
- What can the nurse delegate?
  - What tasks can only the RN perform?
  - What client care responsibilities can the nurse delegate to other health care team members (practical nurses [PNs] and assistive personnel [APs])?

Use time-saving strategies and avoid time wasters. (1.2)
- **Good time management:**
  - Facilitates greater productivity.
  - Decreases work-related stress.
  - Helps ensure the provision of quality client care.
  - Enhances satisfaction with care provided.

1.2 Time management examples

Time savers

Documenting nursing interventions as soon as possible after completion to facilitate accurate and thorough documentation

Grouping activities that are to be performed on the same client or are in close physical proximity to prevent unnecessary walking

Estimating how long each activity will take and planning accordingly

Mentally envisioning the procedure to be performed and gathering all equipment prior to entering the client's room

Taking time to plan care and taking priorities into consideration

Delegating activities to other staff when client care workload is beyond what can be handled by one nurse

Enlisting the aid of other staff when a team approach is more efficient than an individual approach

Completing more difficult or strenuous tasks when energy level is high

Avoiding interruptions and graciously but assertively saying "no" to unreasonable or poorly-timed requests for help

Setting a realistic standard for completion of care and level of performance within the constraints of assignment and resources

Completing one task before beginning another task

Breaking large tasks into smaller tasks to make them more manageable

Using an organizational sheet to plan care

Using breaks to socialize with staff

Time wasters

Documenting at the end of the shift all client care provided and assessments done

Making repeated trips to the supply room for equipment

Providing care as opportunity arises regardless of other responsibilities

Missing equipment when preparing to perform a procedure

Failing to plan or managing by crisis

Being reluctant to delegate or under-delegating

Not asking for help when needed or trying to provide all client care independently

Procrastinating: delaying time-consuming, less desirable tasks until late in the shift

Agreeing to help other team members with lower priority tasks when time is already compromised

Setting unrealistic standards for completion of care and level of performance within constraints of assignment and resources

Starting several tasks at once and not completing tasks before starting others

Not addressing low level of skill competency, increasing time on task

Providing care without a written plan

Socializing with staff during client care time

- **Poor time management:**
  - Impairs productivity.
  - Leads to feelings of being overwhelmed and stressed.
  - Increases omission of important tasks.
  - Creates dissatisfaction with care provided.

Time management is a cyclic process.
- Time initially spent developing a plan will save time later and help to avoid management by crisis.
- Set goals and plan care based on established priorities and thoughtful utilization of resources.
- Complete one client care task before beginning the next, starting with the highest priority task.
- Reprioritize remaining tasks based on continual reassessment of client care needs.
- At the end of the day, perform a time analysis and determine if time was used wisely.

TIME MANAGEMENT AND TEAMWORK

- Be cognizant of assistance needed by other health care team members.
- Offer to help when unexpected crises occur.
- Assist other team members with provision of care when experiencing a period of down time.

TIME MANAGEMENT AND SELF-CARE

- Take time for yourself.
- Schedule time for breaks and meals.
- Take physical and mental breaks from work and the unit.

Assigning, delegating, and supervising

Assigning is the process of transferring the authority, accountability, and responsibility of client care to another member of the health care team. QTC

Delegating is the process of transferring the authority and responsibility to another team member to complete a task, while retaining the accountability.

Supervising is the process of directing, monitoring, and evaluating the performance of tasks by another member of the health care team.

Nurses must delegate appropriately and supervise adequately to ensure that clients receive safe, quality care. (1.3) Qs
- Delegation decisions are based on individual client needs, facility policies and job descriptions, state nurse practice acts, and professional standards. The nurse should consider legal/ethical concerns when assigning and delegating.
- The nurse leader should recognize limitations and use available information and resources to make the best possible decisions at the time. The nurse must remember that it is their responsibility to ensure that clients receive safe, effective nursing care even in tasks delegated to others.
- Nurses must follow the ANA codes of standards in delegating and assigning tasks.

ASSIGNING

Assigning is performed in a downward or lateral manner with regard to members of the health care team.

CLIENT FACTORS

- Condition of the client and level of care needed
- Specific care needs (cardiac monitoring, mechanical ventilation)
- Need for special precautions (isolation precautions, fall precautions, seizure precautions)
- Procedures requiring a significant time commitment (extensive dressing changes or wound care)

HEALTH CARE TEAM FACTORS

- Knowledge and skill level of team members
- Amount of supervision necessary
- Staffing mix (RNs, PNs, APs)
- Nurse-to-client ratio
- Experience with similar clients
- Familiarity of staff member with unit

ADDITIONAL FACTORS

When a nurse receives an unsafe assignment, they should take the following actions.
- Bring the unsafe assignment to the attention of the scheduling/charge nurse and negotiate a new assignment.
- If no resolution is arrived at, take the concern up the chain of command.
- If a satisfactory resolution is still not arrived at, the nurse should file a written protest to the assignment (an assignment despite objection [ADO] or document of practice situation [DOPS]) with the appropriate administrator.
- Failure to accept the assignment without following the proper channels can be considered client abandonment.

MAKING CLIENT ROOM ASSIGNMENTS

The nurse should consider client age and diagnosis, as well as client safety, comfort, privacy, and infection control needs when planning client room assignments. QPCC

Private rooms
Private rooms are required for clients who have an infectious disease that requires airborne precautions, or clients who require a protective environment.

Private rooms are preferred for clients who are on droplet and contact precautions. These clients can cohort if no private rooms are available and if all of the following are true.
- The clients have the same active infection with the same micro-organisms.
- The clients remain at least 3 feet away from each other.
- The clients have no other existing infection.

A private room is also preferred for the following clients.
- Client who are agitated
- Client who have dementia and a history of wandering
- Clients who require a quiet environment (those at risk for increased intracranial pressure [stroke, traumatic brain injury])
- Clients who are at risk for sensory overload (those who are having pain, are acutely ill, have invasive tubes [nasogastric, IVs, endotracheal], or have reduced cognitive function [head injury])
- Clients who require privacy (those who are near death)

Other considerations
- A client who is confused or disoriented should be assigned a room away from noise and away from exits.
- Children who are transitioning from a critical care unit to a lower level of care should be assigned a room near the nurses station and with a roommate of similar age.

DELEGATING AND SUPERVISING

A licensed nurse is responsible for providing clear directions when a task is initially delegated and for periodic reassessment and evaluation of the outcome of the task.
- RNs delegate to other RNs, PNs, and APs.
  - RNs must be knowledgeable about the applicable state nurse practice act and regulations regarding the use of PNs and APs.
  - RNs delegate tasks so that they can complete higher level tasks that only RNs can perform. This allows more efficient use of all members of the health care team. Qтc
- PNs can delegate to other PNs and APs.

DELEGATION FACTORS

- Nurses can only delegate tasks appropriate for the skill and education level of the health care team member who is receiving the assignment.
- RNs cannot delegate the nursing process, client education, or tasks that require clinical judgment to PNs or APs.

1.3 The health care team

LICENSED PERSONNEL: Nurses who have completed a course of study, successfully passed either the NCLEX-PN® or NCLEX-RN® exam, and have a nursing license issued by a board of nursing.

ASSISTIVE PERSONNEL: Specifically trained to function in an assistive role to licensed nurses in client care activities.

These individuals can be nursing personnel (certified nursing assistants [CNAs] or certified medical assistants [CMAs]), or they can be non-nursing personnel to whom nursing activities can be delegated (dialysis technicians, monitor technicians, and phlebotomists).

Some health care entities can differentiate between nurse and non-nurse assistive personnel by using the acronym NAP for nursing assistive personnel.

TASK FACTORS

Prior to delegating client care, consider the following.

Predictability of outcome
- Will the completion of the task have a predictable outcome?
- Is it a routine treatment?
- Is it a new treatment?

Potential for harm
- Is there a chance that something negative can happen to the client (risk for bleeding, risk for aspiration)?
- Is the client unstable?

Complexity of care
- Are complex tasks required as a part of the client's care?
- Is the delegatee legally able to perform the task and do they have the skills necessary?

Need for problem solving and innovation
- Is nursing judgment required while performing the task?
- Does it require nursing assessment skills?

Level of interaction with the client
- Is there a need to provide psychosocial support or education during the performance of the task?

DELEGATEE FACTORS

Considerations for selection of an appropriate delegatee include the following.
- Education, training, and experience
- Knowledge and skill to perform the task
- Level of critical thinking required to complete the task
- Ability to communicate with others as it pertains to the task
- Demonstrated competence
- The delegatee's culture
- Agency policies and procedures and licensing legislation (state nurse practice acts)

DELEGATION AND SUPERVISION GUIDELINES

- Use nursing judgment and knowledge related to the scope of practice and the delegatee's skill level when delegating.
- Use the five rights of delegation. (1.4) Qтc
  - What tasks the nurse delegates (right task)
  - Under what circumstances (right circumstance)
  - To whom (right person)
  - What information should be communicated (right direction/communication)
  - How to supervise/evaluate (right supervision/evaluation)

1.4 The five rights of delegation

RIGHT task
RIGHT circumstance
RIGHT person
RIGHT direction and communication
RIGHT supervision and evaluation

1.5 Examples of tasks nurses can delegate to practical nurses and assistive personnel
(provided the facility's policy and state's practice guidelines permit)

TO PN
Monitoring findings (as input to the RN's ongoing assessment)
Reinforcing client teaching from a standard care plan
Performing tracheostomy care
Suctioning
Checking NG tube patency
Administering enteral feedings
Inserting a urinary catheter
Administering medication (excluding IV medication in some states)

TO AP

Activities of daily living (ADLs)	Positioning
Bathing	Routine tasks
Grooming	Bed making
Dressing	Specimen collection
Toileting	Intake and output
Ambulating	Vital signs (for stable clients)
Feeding (without swallowing precautions)	

Right task

- Identify what tasks are appropriate to delegate for each specific client.
- A right task is repetitive, requires little supervision, and is relatively noninvasive for the client.
- Delegate tasks to appropriate levels of team members (PN, AP) based on standards of practice, legal and facility guidelines, and available resources.

RIGHT TASK: Delegate an AP to assist a client who has pneumonia to use a bedpan.

WRONG TASK: Delegate an AP to administer a nebulizer treatment to a client who has pneumonia.

Right circumstance

- Assess the health status and complexity of care required by the client.
- Match the complexity of care demands to the skill level of the health care team member.
- Consider the workload of the team member.

RIGHT CIRCUMSTANCE: Delegate an AP to measure the vital signs of a client who is postoperative and stable.

WRONG CIRCUMSTANCE: Delegate an AP to measure the vital signs of a client who is postoperative and received naloxone to reverse respiratory depression.

Right person

- Assess and verify the competency of the health care team member.
  - The task must be within the team member's scope of practice.
  - The team member must have the necessary competence/training.
- Continually review the performance of the team member and determine care competency.
- Assess team member performance based on standards and, when necessary, take steps to remediate a failure to meet standards.

RIGHT PERSON: Delegate a PN to administer enteral feedings to a client who has a head injury.

WRONG PERSON: Delegate an AP to administer enteral feedings to a client who has a head injury.

Right direction/communication

Communicate either in writing or orally.
- Data that needs to be collected
- Method and timeline for reporting, including when to report concerns/findings
- Specific task(s) to be performed; client-specific instructions
- Expected results, timelines, and expectations for follow-up communication

RIGHT DIRECTION AND COMMUNICATION: Delegate an AP to assist the client in room 312 with a shower before 0900 and to notify the nurse when complete.

WRONG DIRECTION AND COMMUNICATION: Delegate an AP to assist the client in room 312 with morning hygiene.

Right supervision/evaluation Qᴛᴄ

The delegating nurse must:
- Provide supervision, either directly or indirectly (assigning supervision to another licensed nurse).
- Provide clear directions and expectations of the task to be performed (time frames, what to report).
- Monitor performance.
- Provide feedback.
- Intervene if necessary (unsafe clinical practice).
- Evaluate the client and determine if client outcomes were met.
- Evaluate client care tasks and identify needs for quality improvement activities and/or additional resources.

RIGHT SUPERVISION: Delegate the ambulation of a client to an AP. Observe the AP to ensure safe ambulation of the client, and provide positive feedback to the AP after completion of the task.

WRONG SUPERVISION: Delegate the ambulation of a client to an AP without supervision to determine the need for intervention and failing to provide feedback to the AP.

SUPERVISION

Supervision occurs after delegation. A supervisor oversees a staff member's performance of delegated activities and determines if:

- Completion of tasks is on schedule.
- Performance was at a satisfactory level.
- Unexpected findings were documented and reported or addressed.
- Assistance was required to complete assigned tasks in a timely manner.
- Assignment should be re-evaluated and possibly changed.

Staff education

Staff education refers to the nurse's involvement in the orientation, socialization, education, and training of fellow health care workers to ensure the competence of all staff and to help them meet standards set forth by the facility and accrediting bodies. The process of staff education is also referred to as staff development.

- The quality of client care provided is directly related to the education and level of competency of health care providers. Q**EBP**
- The nurse leader has a responsibility in maintaining competent staff.
- Nurse leaders work with a unique, diverse workforce. The nurse should respect and recognize the health care team's diversity. Q**TC**

1.6 Staff education

CHARACTERISTICS	IDENTIFIED/ PROVIDED BY
Involves methods appropriate to learning domain and learning styles of staff.	Peers, unit managers, staff development educators
Initiated in specific situations • New policies or procedures implemented • New equipment becomes available • Educational need identified	Unit managers, staff development educators
Can focus on one-on-one approach	Unit manager, charge nurse, preceptor
Can use "just in time" training to meet immediate needs for client care	Staff members, supervisors
Higher education degree or certification	Staff

ORIENTATION

Orientation helps newly licensed nurses translate the knowledge, skills, and attitudes learned in nursing school into practice.

ORIENTATION TO THE INSTITUTION

- The newly licensed nurse is introduced to the philosophy, mission, and goals of the institution and department.
- Policies and procedures that are based on institutional standards are reviewed.
- Use of and access to the institution's computer system is a significant focus.
- Safety and security protocols are emphasized in relation to the nurse's role.

ORIENTATION TO THE UNIT

- Classroom orientation is usually followed by orientation to the unit by an experienced nurse.
- Preceptors assist in orienting newly licensed nurses to a unit and supervising their performance and acquisition of skills.
- Preceptors are usually assigned to newly licensed nurses for a limited amount of time.
- Mentors can also serve as a newly licensed nurse's preceptor, but their relationship usually lasts longer and focuses more on assumption of the professional role and relationships, as well as socialization to practice.
- Coaches establish a collaborative relationship to help a nurse establish specific individual goals. The relationship is often task-related and typically time limited.

SOCIALIZATION

Socialization is the process by which a person learns a new role and the values and culture of the group within which that role is implemented.

- Successful socialization helps new staff members fit in with already established staff on a client care unit.
- Staff development educators and unit managers can begin this process during interviewing and orientation.
- Nurse preceptors/mentors are frequently used to assist newly licensed nurses with this process on the clinical unit.

EDUCATION AND TRAINING

Staff education, or staff development, is the process by which a staff member gains knowledge and skills. The goal of staff education is to ensure that staff members have and maintain the most current knowledge and skills necessary to meet the needs of clients. (1.6)

Steps in providing educational programs QEBP

1. Identify and respond: Determine the need for knowledge or skill proficiency

2. Analyze: Look for deficiencies, and develop learning objectives to meet the need

3. Research: Resources available to address learning objectives based on evidence–based practice

4. Plan: Program to address objectives using available resources

5. Implement: Program(s) at a time conducive to staff availability; consider online learning modules

6. Evaluate: Use materials and observations to measure behavior changes secondary to learning objectives

Improved nursing ability

An increase in knowledge and competence is the goal of staff education.

Competence is the ability of an employee to meet the requirements of a particular role at an established level of performance. Nurses usually progress through several stages of proficiency as they gain experience in a particular area.

The five stages of nursing ability were identified by Patricia Benner (1984), and are based on level of competence. Level of competence is directly related to length of time in practice and exposure to clinical situations. When nurses move to a new clinical setting that requires acquisition of new skills and knowledge, their level of competence will return to a lower stage. (1.7)

Quality improvement

- Quality improvement (performance improvement, quality control) is the process used to identify and resolve performance deficiencies. Quality improvement includes measuring performance against a set of predetermined standards. In health care, these standards are set by the facility and consider accrediting and professional standards. QQI
- Standards of care should reflect optimal goals and be based on evidence.
- The quality improvement process focuses on assessment of outcomes and determines ways to improve the delivery of quality care. All levels of employees are involved in the quality improvement process.
- The Joint Commission's accreditation standards require institutions to show evidence of quality improvement in order to attain accreditation status.

1.7 Five stages of nursing ability

Novice nurse

Novice nurses can be students or newly licensed nurses who have minimal clinical experience. They approach situations from theoretical perspective relying on context-free facts and established guidelines. Rules govern practice.

Advanced beginner

Most new nurses function at the level of the advanced beginner. They practice independently in the performance of many tasks and can make some clinical judgments. They begin to rely on prior experience to make practice decisions.

Competent nurse

These are usually nurses who have been in practice for 2 to 3 years. They demonstrate increasing levels of skill and proficiency and clinical judgment. They exhibit the ability to organize and plan care using abstract and analytical thinking. They can anticipate the long-term outcomes of personal actions.

Proficient nurse

These are nurses who have a significant amount of experience upon which to base their practice. Enhanced observational abilities allow nurses to be able to conceptualize situations more holistically. Well-developed critical thinking and decision-making skills allow nurses to recognize and respond to unexpected changes.

Expert nurse

Expert nurses have garnered a wealth of experience so they can view situations holistically and process information efficiently. They make decisions using an advanced level of intuition and analytical ability. They do not need to rely on rules to comprehend a situation and take action.

Source: http://www.scribd.com/doc/27103958/Benner-Theory-Novice-to-Expert

QUALITY IMPROVEMENT PROCESS

The quality improvement process begins with identification of standards and outcome indicators based on evidence.

Outcome (clinical) indicators reflect desired client outcomes related to the standard under review. QEBP

Structure indicators reflect the setting in which care is provided and the available human and material resources.

Process indicators reflect how client care is provided and are established by policies and procedures (clinical practice guidelines).

Benchmarks are goals that are set to determine at what level the outcome indicators should be met.

While process indicators provide important information about how a procedure is being carried out, an outcome indicator measures whether that procedure is effective in meeting the desired benchmark. For example, the use of incentive spirometers in postoperative clients can be determined to be 92% (process indicator), but the rate of postoperative pneumonia can be determined to be 8% (outcome indicator). If the benchmark is set at 5%, the benchmark for that outcome indicator is not being met and the structure and process variables need to be analyzed to identify potential areas for improvement.

STEPS IN THE QUALITY IMPROVEMENT PROCESS

A standard is developed and approved by a facility committee.

- Standards are made available to employees by way of policies and procedures.
- Quality issues are identified by the staff, management, or risk management department.
- An interprofessional team is developed to review the issue.
- The current state of structure and process related to the issue is analyzed.
- Data collection methods are determined.
  - Quantitative methods are primarily used in the data collection process, although client interview is also an option.
- Data is collected, analyzed, and compared with the established benchmark.
- If the benchmark is not met, possible influencing factors are determined. A root cause analysis can be done to critically assess all factors that influence the issue. A root cause analysis: Q EBP
  - Focuses on variables that surround the consequence of an action or occurrence.
  - Is commonly done for sentinel events (client death, client care resulting in serious physical injury) but can also be done as part of the quality improvement process.
  - Investigates the consequence and possible causes.
  - Analyzes the possible causes and relationships that can exist.
  - Determines additional influences at each level of relationship.
  - Determines the root cause or causes.
- Potential solutions or corrective actions are analyzed and one is selected for implementation.
- Educational or corrective action is implemented.
- The issue is reevaluated at a preestablished time to determine the efficacy of the solution or corrective action.

Core measures

National standardized measures are developed by the Joint Commission to improve client outcomes. It is used to measure client outcomes and provides information to support accreditation of hospitals.

Core measures developed include stroke, venous thromboembolism, heart failure, acute myocardial infarction, and substance use.

Audits

Audits can produce valuable quantitative data.

Types of audits

- Structure audits evaluate the influence of elements that exist separate from or outside of the client-staff interaction.
- Process audits review how care was provided and assume a relationship exists between nurses and the quality of care provided.
- Outcome audits determine what results, if any, occurred as a result of the nursing care provided.
  - Some outcomes are influenced by aspects of care (the quality of medical care, the level of commitment of managerial staff, and the characteristics of the facility's policies and procedures).
  - Nursing-sensitive outcomes are those that are directly affected by the quality of nursing care. Examples include client fall rates and the incidence of nosocomial infections.

Timing of audits

- Retrospective audits occur after the client receives care.
- Concurrent audits occur while the client is receiving care.
- Prospective audits predict how future client care will be affected by the current level of services.

NURSE'S ROLE IN QUALITY IMPROVEMENT

- Serve as unit representative on committees developing policies and procedures.
- Use reliable resources for information (Centers for Disease Control and Prevention, professional journals, evidenced-based research). Q EBP
- Enhance knowledge and understanding of the facility's policies and procedures.
- Provide client care consistent with these policies and procedures.
- Document client care thoroughly and according to facility guidelines.
- Participate in the collection of information/data related to staff's adherence to selected policy or procedure.
- Assist with analysis of the information/data.
- Compare results with the established benchmark.
- Make a judgment about performance in regard to the findings.
- Assist with provision of education or training necessary to improve the performance of staff.
- Act as a role model by practicing in accordance with the established standard.
- Assist with re-evaluation of staff performance by collection of information/data at a specified time.

Nursing strategies to promote evidence-based approach to client care

- Remain aware of current trends in research.
- Incorporate evidence into clinical practice.
- Question traditional nursing practice to promote change.
- Collaborate with other disciplines to enrich practice.
- Use the PICO model (population, intervention, comparison, and outcome) to find current evidence to guide best practice.

Quality improvement tools for tracking outcomes

Structured care methodologies are used to track variances, measure outcomes, improve quality, and facilitate best practices.

Standards of care: Baseline of quality care a client should receive

Algorithms: Series of progressive treatment based on client response (advanced cardiac life support)

Critical or clinical pathway: Projected path of treatment based on a set time frame for clients who have comparable diagnoses

Protocols: Standard guidelines for a specific intervention (stroke protocol)

Guidelines: Evidence-based information to provide quality care and improve outcomes

Performance appraisal, peer review, and disciplinary action

A performance appraisal is the process by which a supervisor evaluates an employee's performance in relation to the job description for that employee's position as well as other expectations the facility can have.

- Performance appraisals are done at regular intervals and can be more frequent for new employees.
- Performance expectations should be based on the standards set forth in a job description and written in objective terms.
- Performance appraisals allow nurses the opportunity to discuss personal goals with the unit manager as well as to receive feedback regarding level of performance. Performance appraisals can also be used as a motivational tool.
- Deficiencies identified during a performance appraisal or reported by coworkers might need to be addressed in a disciplinary manner.

PERFORMANCE APPRAISAL AND PEER REVIEW

- A formal system for conducting performance appraisals should be in place and used consistently. Performance appraisal tools should reflect the staff member's job description and can be based on various types of scales or surveys.
- Various sources of data should be collected to ensure an unbiased and thorough evaluation of an employee's performance.
  - Data should be collected over time and not just represent isolated incidents.
  - Actual observed behavior should be documented/used as evidence of satisfactory or unsatisfactory performance. These can be called anecdotal notes and are kept in the unit manager or equivalent position's files.
  - Peers can be a valuable source of data. Peer review is the evaluation of a colleague's practice by another peer. Peer review should:
    - Begin with an orientation of staff to the peer review process, their professional responsibility in regard to promoting growth of colleagues, and the disposition of data collected.
    - Focus on the peer's performance in relation to the job description or an appraisal tool that is based on institutional standards.
    - Be shared with the peer and usually the manager.
    - Be only part of the data used when completing a staff member's performance appraisal.
  - The employee should be given the opportunity to provide input into the evaluation.
- The unit manager should host the performance appraisal review in a private setting at a time conducive to the staff member's attendance. The unit manager should review the data with the staff member and provide the opportunity for feedback. Personal goals of the staff member are discussed and documented, including avenues for attainment. Staff members who do not agree with the unit manager's evaluation of their performance should have the opportunity to make written comments on the evaluation form and appeal the rating.

DISCIPLINARY ACTION

- Deficiencies identified during a performance appraisal or the course of employment should be presented in writing, and corrective action should be based on institutional policy regarding disciplinary actions and/or termination of employment. Evidence regarding the deficiency must support such a claim. **(1.8)**
- Some offenses (mistreatment of a client or use of alcohol or other substances while working) warrant immediate dismissal. Lesser infractions should follow a stepwise manner, giving the staff member the opportunity to correct unacceptable behavior.
- Staff members who witness an inappropriate action by a coworker should report the infraction up the chain of command. At the time of the infraction, this might be the charge nurse. The unit manager should also be notified, and written documentation by the manager is placed in the staff member's permanent file.

Conflict resolution

Conflict is the result of opposing thoughts, ideas, feelings, perceptions, behaviors, values, opinions, or actions between individuals.

- Conflict is an inevitable part of professional, social, and personal life and can have constructive or destructive results. Nurses must understand conflict and how to manage it.
- Nurses can use problem-solving and negotiation strategies to prevent a problem from evolving into a conflict. Qtc
- Lack of conflict can create organizational stasis, while too much conflict can be demoralizing, produce anxiety, and contribute to burnout.
- Conflict can disrupt working relationships and create a stressful atmosphere.
- If conflict exists to the level that productivity and quality of care are compromised, the unit manager must attempt to identify the origin of the conflict and attempt to resolve it.

Common causes of conflict

- Ineffective communication
- Unclear expectations of team members in their various roles
- Poorly defined or actualized organizational structure
- Conflicts of interest and variance in standards
- Incompatibility of individuals
- Management or staffing changes
- Diversity related to age, gender, race, or ethnicity

CATEGORIES OF CONFLICT

INTRAPERSONAL CONFLICT

Occurs within the person and can involve internal struggle related to contradictory values or wants.

> Example: A nurse wants to move up on the career ladder but is finding that time with their family is subsequently compromised.

INTERPERSONAL CONFLICT

Occurs between two or more people with differing values, goals, or beliefs.

- Interpersonal conflict in the health care setting involves disagreement among nurses, clients, family members, and within a health care team. Bullying and incivility in the workplace are forms of interpersonal conflict.
- This is a significant issue in nursing, especially in relation to new nurses, who bring new personalities and perspectives to various health care settings.
- Interpersonal conflict contributes to burnout and work-related stress.

> Example: A new nurse is given a client assignment that is heavier than those of other nurses, and when the new nurse asks for help, it is denied.

INTERGROUP CONFLICT

Occurs between two or more groups of individuals, departments, or organizations and can be caused by a new policy or procedure, a change in leadership, or a change in organizational structure.

> Example: There is confusion as to whether it is the responsibility of the nursing unit or dietary department to pass meal trays to clients.

STAGES OF CONFLICT

Five stages of conflict exist. If the nurse manager is familiar with the stages there is an increased chance that the conflict can be resolved effectively.

STAGE 1: LATENT CONFLICT

The actual conflict has not yet developed; however, factors are present that have a high likelihood of causing conflict to occur.

> Example: A new scheduling policy is implemented within the organization. The nurse manager should recognize that change is a common cause of conflict.

STAGE 2: PERCEIVED CONFLICT

A party perceives that a problem is present, though an actual conflict might not actually exist.

> Example: A nurse perceives that a nurse manager is unfair with scheduling. The nurse might not be aware that, in reality, it is only because the nurse manager misunderstood the nurse's scheduling request.

STAGE 3: FELT CONFLICT

Those involved begin to feel an emotional response to the conflict.

> Example: A nurse feels anger towards the nurse manager after finding out that they are scheduled to work two holidays in a row.

STAGE 4: MANIFEST CONFLICT

The parties involved are aware of the conflict and action is taken. Actions at this stage can be positive and strive towards conflict resolution, or they can be negative and include debating, competing, or withdrawal of one or more parties from the situation.

> Example: The nurse manager and nurses on a unit agree that the current scheduling system is causing a conflict and agree to work together to come up with a solution.

STAGE 5: CONFLICT AFTERMATH

Conflict aftermath is the completion of the conflict process and can be positive or negative.

> Example: Positive conflict aftermath: the nurse manager and nurses on a unit are satisfied with the newly revised scheduling system and feel valued for being included in the conflict resolution process.

> Example: Negative conflict aftermath: the nurse manager and nurses are unable to come up with a scheduling solution that meets the needs of both parties. They agree to continue with the current system; however, tensions still remain, increasing the risk of a recurrence of the conflict.

CONFLICT RESOLUTION STRATEGIES

PROBLEM-SOLVING

- Open communication among staff and between staff and clients can help defray the need for conflict resolution. Qᴛᴄ
- When potential sources of conflict exist, the use of open communication and problem-solving strategies are effective tools to de-escalate the situation.

Actions nurses can take to promote open communication and de-escalate conflicts

- Use "I" statements, and remember to focus on the problem, not on personal differences.
- Listen carefully to what others are saying, and try to understand their perspective.
- Move a conflict that is escalating to a private location or postpone the discussion until a later time to give everyone a chance to regain control of their emotions.
- Share ground rules with participants. For example, everyone is to be treated with respect, only one person can speak at a time, and everyone should have a chance to speak.

Steps of the problem-solving process

Identify the problem. State it in objective terms, minimizing emotional overlay.

Discuss possible solutions. Brainstorming solutions as a group can stimulate new solutions to old problems. Encourage individuals to think creatively, beyond simple solutions.

Analyze identified solutions. The potential pros and cons of each possible solution should be discussed in an attempt to narrow down the number of viable solutions.

Select a solution. Based on this analysis, select a solution for implementation.

Implement the selected solution. A procedure and timeline for implementation should accompany the implementation of the selected solution.

Evaluate the solution's ability to resolve the original problem. The outcomes surrounding the new solution should be evaluated according to the predetermined timeline. The solution should be given adequate time to become established as a new routine before it is evaluated. If the solution is deemed unsuccessful, the problem-solving process will need to be reinstituted and the problem discussed again.

1.8 Steps in progressive discipline

First infraction
Informal reprimand
Manager and employee meet
Discuss the issue
Suggestions for improvement/correction

Second infraction
Written warning
Manager meets with employee to distribute written warning
Review of specific rules/policy violations
Discussion of potential consequences if infractions continue

Third infraction
Employee placed on suspension with or without pay. Time away from work gives the employee opportunity to:
Examine the issues
Consider alternatives

Fourth infraction
Employee termination
Follows after multiple warnings have been given and employee continues to violate rules and policies

NEGOTIATION

- Negotiation is the process by which interested parties:
  - Resolve ongoing conflicts.
  - Agree on steps to take.
  - Bargain to protect individual or collective interests.
  - Pursue outcomes that benefit mutual interests.
- Most nurses use negotiation on a daily basis.
- Negotiation can involve the use of several conflict resolution strategies.
- The focus is on a win-win solution or a win/lose-win/lose solution in which both parties win and lose a portion of their original objectives. Each party agrees to give up something and the emphasis is on accommodating differences rather than similarities between parties.

Example

One nurse offers to care for Client A today if the other will care for Client B tomorrow.

Strategy: Avoiding/Withdrawing
- Both parties know there is a conflict, but they refuse to face it or work toward a resolution.
- Can be appropriate for minor conflicts, when one party holds more power than the other party, or if the issue can work itself out over time.
- Because the conflict remains, it can surface again at a later date and escalate over time.
- This is usually a lose-lose solution.

Strategy: Smoothing
- One party attempts to "smooth" another party by trying to satisfy the other party.
- Often used to preserve or maintain a peaceful work environment.
- The focus can be on what is agreed upon, leaving conflict largely unresolved.
- This is usually a lose-lose solution.

Strategy: Competing/Coercing
- One party pursues a desired solution at the expense of others.
- Managers can use this when a quick or unpopular decision must be made.
- The party who loses something can experience anger, aggravation, and a desire for retribution.
- This is usually a win-lose solution.

Strategy: Cooperating/Accommodating
- One party sacrifices something, allowing the other party to get what it wants. This is the opposite of competing.
- The original problem might not actually be resolved.
- The solution can contribute to future conflict.
- This is a lose-win solution.

Strategy: Compromising/Negotiating
- Each party gives up something.
- To consider this a win/lose-win/lose solution, both parties must give up something equally important. If one party gives up more than the other, it can become a win-lose solution.

Strategy: Collaborating
- Both parties set aside their original individual goals and work together to achieve a new common goal.
- Requires mutual respect, positive communication, and shared decision-making between parties.
- This is a win-win solution.

Example

An experienced nurse on a urology unit arrives to work on the night shift. The unit manager immediately asks the nurse to float to a pediatrics unit because the hospital census is high and they are understaffed. The nurse has always maintained a positive attitude when asked to work on another medical-surgical unit but states they do not feel comfortable in the pediatric setting. The manager insists the nurse is the most qualified.

Strategy: Avoiding/Withdrawing/Smoothing
The nurse basically cannot use these strategies due to the immediacy of the situation. The assignment cannot be simply avoided or smoothed over; it must be accepted or rejected.

Strategy: Competing/Coercing
- If the nurse truly feels unqualified to work on the pediatric unit, then this approach can be appropriate: the nurse must win and the manager must lose.
- Although risking termination by refusing the assignment, the nurse should take an assertive approach and inform the manager that pediatric clients would be placed at risk.

Strategy: Cooperating/Accommodating
- If the nurse decides to accommodate the manager's request, then the pediatric clients can be at risk for incompetent care.
- Practice liability is another issue for consideration.

Strategy: Compromising/Negotiating
- This approach generally minimizes the losses for all involved while making certain each party gains something.

For example, the nurse might offer to work on another medical-surgical unit if someone from that unit feels comfortable in the pediatric environment.

- Although each party is giving up something (the manager gives in to a different solution and the nurse still has to work on another unit), this sort of compromise can result in a win-win resolution.

Strategy: Collaborating
Both the nurse manager and nurse come to the agreement that providing safe and competent care of the children in the pediatric unit is the common goal. While they might need to compromise/negotiate to address the immediate need, they can collaborate to achieve a solution that avoids this situation in the future.

For example, the nurse might agree to orient to the pediatric unit in order to become competent for future assignments and the nurse manager can enlist the services of a staffing agency that provides pediatric nurses on an as needed basis.

ASSERTIVE COMMUNICATION

- Use of assertive communication can be necessary during conflict negotiation.
- Assertive communication allows expression in direct, honest, and nonthreatening ways that do not infringe upon the rights of others.
- It is a communication style that acknowledges and deals with conflict, recognizes others as equals, and provides a direct statement of feelings.

Elements of assertive communication

- Selecting an appropriate location for verbal exchange
- Maintenance of eye contact
- Establishing trust
- Being sensitive to cultural needs
- Speaking using "I" statements and including affective elements of the situation
- Avoiding "you" statements that can indicate blame
- Stating concerns using open, honest, direct statements
- Conveying empathy
- Focusing on the behavior or issue of conflict and avoiding personal attacks
- Concluding with a statement that describes a fair solution

GRIEVANCES

- A grievance is a wrong perceived by an employee based on a feeling of unfair treatment that is considered grounds for a formal complaint.
- Grievances that cannot be satisfactorily resolved between the parties involved can require management by a third party.
- Facilities have a formal grievance policy that should be followed when a conflict cannot be resolved.
- The steps of an institution's grievance procedure should be outlined in the grievance policy.

Typical steps of the grievance process

- Started at the first level of management and continued up the chain of command as needed
- Formal hearing if the issue is not resolved at a lower level
- Professional mediation if a solution is not reached during a formal hearing

Resource management

Resource management includes budgeting and resource allocation. Human, financial, and material resources must be considered.

- Budgeting is usually the responsibility of the unit manager, but staff nurses can be asked to provide input.
- Resource allocation is a responsibility of the unit manager as well as every practicing nurse.
- Providing cost-effective client care should not compromise quality of care.

Resources (supplies, equipment, personnel) are critical to accomplishing the goals and objectives of a health care facility, so it is essential for nurses to understand how to effectively manage resources. Qᵍⁱ

COST-EFFECTIVE CARE

Cost-containment

Strategies that promote efficient and competent client care while also producing needed revenues for the continued productivity of the organization

> Example: The use of managed care strives to provide clients with a plan designed to meet the needs of their individual medical problem while eliminating the unnecessary use of resources or extended hospital stays.

Cost-effective

Strategies that achieve optimal results in relation to the money spent to achieve those results. In other words, cost-effective means "getting your money's worth."

> Example: Spending increased money on staff training for transmission-based precautions, resulting in the increased and effective use of PPE for client care. These actions have the end result of a decrease in infection transmission and an overall savings in the cost of caring for clients who would have acquired these infections.

COST-EFFECTIVE CARE STRATEGIES

Providing clients with needed education to decrease or eliminate future medical costs associated with future complications

Example: Teaching a client who has a new diagnosis of diabetes mellitus how to adjust the dosage of insulin depending on activity level, reducing the risk of hypoglycemia resulting in the need for medical care.

Promoting the use of evidence-based care, resulting in improved client care outcomes

Example: Implementing the use of evidence-based techniques to care for clients who have indwelling catheters, resulting in a decreased incidence of catheter-acquired urinary tract infections.

Promoting cost-effective resource management

Example: Using all levels of personnel to their fullest when making assignments. Delegating effectively to members of the nursing care team.

Example: Providing necessary equipment and properly charging clients.

Example: Returning uncontaminated, unused equipment to the appropriate department for credit.

Example: Using equipment properly to prevent wastage.

Example: Providing training to staff unfamiliar with equipment.

Example: Returning equipment (IV pumps) to the proper department (central service, central distribution) as soon as it is no longer needed. This action will prevent further cost to clients.

Active Learning Scenario

A nurse manager is discussing emotional intelligence with the charge nurses within the facility. What information should the manager include in this discussion? Use the Active Learning Template: Basic Concept to complete this item.

RELATED CONTENT: Define emotional intelligence.

UNDERLYING PRINCIPLES: Identify at least three characteristics of an emotionally intelligent leader.

Active Learning Scenario Key

Using the Active Learning Template: Basic Concept
RELATED CONTENT: Emotional intelligence is the ability of an individual to perceive and manage the emotions of self and others.
UNDERLYING PRINCIPLES
- Insight into the emotions of members of the team
- Understands the perspective of others
- Encourages constructive criticism and is open to new ideas
- Able to maintain focus while multitasking
- Manages emotions and channels them in a positive direction, which in turn helps the team accomplish its goals
- Committed to the delivery of high-quality client care
- Refrains from judgment in controversial or emotionally-charged situations until facts are gathered

Ⓝ *NCLEX® Connection: Management of Care, Concepts of Management*

1. A nurse enters the room of a client and finds the client lying on the floor. Which of the following actions should the nurse take first?

   A. Call the provider.

   B. Ask a staff member for assistance getting the client back in bed.

   C. Inspect the client for injuries.

   D. Instruct the client to ask for help if they need to get out of bed.

2. An RN on a medical-surgical unit is making assignments at the beginning of the shift. Which of the following tasks should the nurse delegate to the PN?

   A. Obtain vital signs for a client who is 2 hr postprocedure following a cardiac catheterization.

   B. Administer a unit of packed red blood cells (RBCs) to a client who has cancer.

   C. Instruct a client who is scheduled for discharge in the performance of wound care.

   D. Develop a plan of care for a newly admitted client who has pneumonia.

3. A PN ending their shift reports to the RN that a newly hired AP has not calculated the intake and output for several clients. Which of the following actions should the RN take?

   A. Complete an incident report.

   B. Delegate this task to the PN.

   C. Ask the AP if they need assistance.

   D. Notify the nurse manager.

4. A nurse manager is developing an orientation plan for newly licensed nurses. Which of the following information should the manager include in the plan? (Select all that apply.)

   A. Skill proficiency

   B. Assignment to a preceptor

   C. Budgetary principles

   D. Computerized charting

   E. Socialization into unit culture

   F. Facility policies and procedures

5. A nurse manager is providing information about the audit process to members of the nursing team. Which of the following information should the nurse manager include? (Select all that apply.)

   A. A structure audit evaluates the setting and resources available to provide care.

   B. An outcome audit evaluates the results of the nursing care provided.

   C. A root cause analysis is indicated when a sentinel event occurs.

   D. Retrospective audits are conducted while the client is receiving care.

   E. After data collection is completed, it is compared to a benchmark.

6. A nurse is participating in a quality improvement study of a procedure frequently performed on the unit. Which of the following information will provide data regarding the efficacy of the procedure?

   A. Frequency with which procedure is performed

   B. Client satisfaction with performance of procedure

   C. Incidence of complications related to procedure

   D. Accurate documentation of how procedure was performed

7. A nurse is hired to replace a staff member who has resigned. After working on the unit for several weeks, the nurse notices that the unit manager does not intervene when there is conflict between team members, even when it escalates. Which of the following conflict resolution strategies is the unit manager demonstrating?

   A. Avoidance

   B. Smoothing

   C. Cooperating

   D. Negotiating

Application Exercises Key

1. A. Notify the provider to determine whether the client needs further examination and treatment, but there is another action to take first.
   B. Seek assistance in returning the client to bed to prevent further harm to the client, but there is another action to take first.
   C. **CORRECT:** The first action to take using the nursing process is to assess the client in order to determine which interventions the client will need.
   D. Instruct the client to ask for help before getting out of bed to help prevent future falls, but there is another action to take first.

   Ⓝ *NCLEX® Connection: Management of Care, Establishing Priorities*

2. A. **CORRECT:** It is within the scope of practice of the PN to monitor a client who is 2 hr postprocedure for a cardiac catheterization, because this client is considered stable.
   B. The RN is responsible for administering blood components, including packed RBCs, because this outside of the scope of practice for the PN.
   C. The RN is responsible for client education. It is within the scope of practice of the PN to reinforce but not provide initial client education.
   D. The RN is responsible for developing a plan of care for a client. It is within the scope of practice for the PN to suggest additions to but not develop the plan of care.

   Ⓝ *NCLEX® Connection: Management of Care, Assignment, Delegation and Supervision*

3. A. An incident report is indicated when a critical incident has occurred. It is not necessary to complete an incident report in this situation.
   B. Do not redelegate this task.
   C. **CORRECT:** Find out what the AP knows about performing the task and provide education for the AP if indicated.
   D. The RN is capable of handling the situation. It is not necessary to notify the nurse manager.

   Ⓝ *NCLEX® Connection: Management of Care, Assignment, Delegation and Supervision*

4. A. **CORRECT:** The purpose of orientation is to assist the newly licensed nurse to transition from the role of student to the role of employee and licensed nurse. Include evaluation of skill proficiency and provide additional instruction as indicated.
   B. **CORRECT:** The purpose of orientation is to assist the newly licensed nurse to transition from the role of student to the role of employee and licensed nurse. Include assignment of a preceptor to ease the transition of the newly licensed nurse.
   C. Budgetary principles are an administrative skill that is usually the responsibility of the unit manager.
   D. **CORRECT:** The purpose of orientation is to assist the newly licensed nurse to transition from the role of student to the role of employee and licensed nurse. Include computerized charting, which is an essential skill for the newly licensed nurse.
   E. **CORRECT:** The purpose of orientation is to assist the newly licensed nurse to transition from the role of student to the role of employee and licensed nurse. Include socialization to the unit as a way to ease the transition of the newly licensed nurse.
   F. **CORRECT:** The purpose of orientation is to assist the newly licensed nurse to transition from the role of student to the role of employee and licensed nurse. Include information about facility policies and procedures, which is essential information for the newly licensed nurse.

   Ⓝ *NCLEX® Connection: Management of Care, Concepts of Management*

5. A. **CORRECT:** A structure audit evaluates the setting in which care is provided and includes resources (equipment and staffing levels).
   B. **CORRECT:** An outcome audit evaluates the effectiveness of nursing care. It should include observable data (infection rates among clients).
   C. **CORRECT:** A root cause analysis is indicated when a sentinel event occurs. A sentinel event is a serious problem (injury to or death of a client). Immediate investigation of the problem is indicated. The health care team can use root cause analysis to study the problem and take measures to prevent recurrence.
   D. Retrospective audits are conducted when the client is no longer receiving care.
   E. **CORRECT:** The benchmark is set at the beginning of the process and then it is compared to the data after collection is completed.

   Ⓝ *NCLEX® Connection: Management of Care, Performance Improvement (Quality Improvement)*

6. A. The frequency with which the procedure is performed is important. The team can take the frequency in which the procedure is performed under consideration in the planning process, but this information does not address the efficacy of the procedure.
   B. The team should take client satisfaction under consideration in the planning process, but this information does not address the efficacy of the procedure.
   C. **CORRECT:** The incidence of complications related to the procedure is an outcome measure directly related to the efficacy of the procedure.
   D. The team can take accuracy of documentation under consideration in the planning process, but this information does not address the efficacy of the procedure.

   Ⓝ *NCLEX® Connection: Management of Care, Performance Improvement (Quality Improvement)*

7. A. **CORRECT:** The goal in resolving conflict is a win-win situation. The unit manager is using an ineffective strategy, avoidance, to deal with this conflict. Although the unit manager is aware of the conflict, they are not attempting to resolve it.
   B. The goal in resolving conflict is a win-win solution. When smoothing is used, one person attempts to "smooth" the other party and/or point out areas in which the parties agree. This is typically a lose-lose solution.
   C. The goal in resolving a conflict is a win-win solution. When cooperating is used, one party allows the other party to win. This is a lose-win solution.
   D. The goal in resolving a conflict is a win-win solution. When negotiating is used, each party gives up something. If one party gives up more than the other, this can become a win-lose solution.

   Ⓝ *NCLEX® Connection: Management of Care, Concepts of Management*

When reviewing the following chapter, keep in mind the relevant topics and tasks of the NCLEX outline, in particular:

Management of Care

CASE MANAGEMENT: Explore resources available to assist the client with achieving or maintaining independence.

CLIENT RIGHTS

Recognize the client's right to refuse treatment/procedures.

Advocate for client rights and needs.

COLLABORATION WITH INTERDISCIPLINARY TEAM

Review plan of care to ensure continuity across disciplines.

Identify significant information to report to other disciplines.

CONCEPTS OF MANAGEMENT: Act as liaison between the client and others.

CONTINUITY OF CARE

Use documents to record and communicate client information.

Provide and receive hand off care (report) on assigned clients.

REFERRALS: Identify community resources for the client.

CHAPTER 2 Coordinating Client Care

One of the primary roles of nursing is the coordination and management of client care in collaboration with the health care team. In so doing, high-quality health care is provided as clients move through the health care system in a cost-effective and time-efficient manner. Qᴛᴄ

To effectively coordinate client care, a nurse must have an understanding of collaboration with the interprofessional team, principles of case management, continuity of care (including consultations, referrals, transfers, and discharge planning), and motivational principles to encourage and empower self, staff, colleagues, and other members of the interprofessional team.

COLLABORATION WITH THE INTERPROFESSIONAL TEAM

An interprofessional team is a group of health care professionals from various disciplines. Collaboration involves discussion of client care issues in making health care decisions, especially for clients who have multiple problems. The specialized knowledge and skills of each discipline are used in the development of an interprofessional plan of care that addresses multiple problems. Nurses should recognize that the collaborative efforts of the interprofessional team allow the achievement of results that a team member would be incapable of accomplishing alone.

- Nurse–provider collaboration should be fostered to create a climate of mutual respect and collaborative practice.
- Collaboration occurs among different levels of nurses and nurses with different areas of expertise.
- Collaboration should also occur between the interprofessional team, the client, and the client's family/significant others when an interprofessional plan of care is being developed.
- Collaboration is a form of conflict resolution that results in a win–win solution for both the client and health care team.

NURSE QUALITIES FOR EFFECTIVE COLLABORATION

- Good communication skills
- Assertiveness
- Conflict negotiation skills
- Leadership skills
- Professional presence
- Decision-making and critical thinking

THE NURSE'S ROLE

- Coordinate the interprofessional team.
- Have a holistic understanding of the client, the client's health care needs, and the health care system.
- Provide the opportunity for care to be provided with continuity over time and across disciplines.
- Provide the client with the opportunity to be a partner in the development of the plan of care.
- Provide information during rounds and interprofessional team meetings regarding the status of the client's health.
- Provide an avenue for the initiation of a consultation related to a specific health care issue.
- Provide a link to postdischarge resources that might need a referral.

VARIABLES THAT AFFECT COLLABORATION

Hierarchical influence on decision-making

Decision-making is also influenced by the facility hierarchy.
- In a centralized hierarchy, nurses at the top of the organizational chart make most of the decisions.
- In a decentralized hierarchy, staff nurses who provide direct client care are included in the decision-making process. Large organizations benefit from the use of decentralized decision-making because managers at the top of the hierarchy do not have firsthand knowledge of unit-level challenges or problems. Decentralized decision-making promotes job satisfaction among staff nurses.

Behavioral change strategies

Although bombarded with constant change, members of the interprofessional team can be resistant to change. Three strategies a manager can use to promote change are the rational-empirical, normative-reeducative, and the power-coercive. Often the manager uses a combination of these strategies.

RATIONAL-EMPIRICAL: The manager provides factual information to support the change. Used when resistance to change is minimal.

NORMATIVE-REEDUCATIVE: The manager focuses on interpersonal relationships to promote change.

POWER-COERCIVE: The manager uses rewards to promote change. Used when individuals are highly resistant to change.

Planned change

Planned change is important in health care because it enables the interprofessional team to replace unproven methods with evidence-based ones.
- Planned change might be a proactive way to improve care quality. Change might also be required by a regulatory board.
- Variables that affect whether change can fully take place include individual and organizational willingness, competing demands, and whether the change is meaningful.
- Changes in technology are more readily accepted than social change.
- Include people who will be affected by the change in the planning process to decrease resistance.

Lewin's change theory

Lewin's change theory is a common model for promoting planned change, which has three stages.
- Unfreezing: Need for change is identified or created.
- Change/Movement: Strategies (driving forces) that overcome resistance to change (restraining forces) are identified and implemented.
- Refreezing: The change is integrated and the system is re-stabilized.

Lewin's theory has been adapted into a stages of change model for individual change, with five stages:
- Precontemplation: No intent to change is present or has been considered.
- Contemplation: The individual considers adopting a change.
- Preparation: The individual intends to implement the change in the near future.
- Action: The individual implements the change.
- Maintenance: The individual continues the new behavior without relapse.

Stages of team formation

Teams typically work through a group formation process before reaching peak performance.

FORMING: Members of the team get to know each other. The leader defines tasks for the team and offers direction.

STORMING: Conflict arises, and team members begin to express polarized views. The team establishes rules, and members begin to take on various roles.

NORMING: The team establishes rules. Members show respect for one another and begin to accomplish some of the tasks.

PERFORMING: The team focuses on accomplishment of tasks.

Generational differences team members

Generational differences influence the value system of the members of an interprofessional team and can affect how members function within the team. Generational differences can be challenging for members of a team, but working with individuals from different generations also can bring strength to the team.
- Veterans (Silent Generation, Traditionals): Born 1925 to 1942
- Baby Boomers: Born 1942 to early 1960s
- Generation X: Born mid-1960s to early 1980s
- Generation Y (Millennial): Born mid-1980s to 2000
- Generation Z (Homelanders): Born after 2001

MAGNET RECOGNITION PROGRAM

The American Nurses Credentialing Center awards Magnet Recognition to health care facilities that provide high-quality client care and attract and retain well-qualified nurses. The term magnet is used to recognize the facility's power to draw nurses to the facility and to retain them. Qoi
- Facilities must create a culture that uses 14 foundational forces of magnetism and model five key components, which include the following.
  - Empirical data showing quality care results
  - Development of innovation, improvements, or generation of new knowledge
  - Exemplary nursing practice
  - A culture of empowerment
  - Transformational leadership
- The facility must submit documentation to the American Nurses Credentialing Center (ANCC) that demonstrates adherence to ANA nurse administrator standards.
- After documentation that the standards have been met, an on-site appraisal is conducted. A facility that meets the standards is awarded magnet status for a 4-year period.

PATHWAY TO EXCELLENCE RECOGNITION

A program of practice standards to promote a positive practice environment using evidence-based standards
- Acute- or long-term care facilities can apply for recognition with this program.
- The Pathway to Excellence designation process includes an application process and adherence to 12 standards of practice, along with an independent survey of the facility.

CASE MANAGEMENT

Case management is the coordination of care provided by an interprofessional team from the time a client starts receiving care until they no longer receive services. Q̇TC

PRINCIPLES OF CASE MANAGEMENT

- Case management focuses on managed care of the client through collaboration of the health care team in acute and post-acute settings.
- The goal of case management is to avoid fragmentation of care and control cost.
- A case manager collaborates with the interprofessional health care team during the assessment of a client's needs and subsequent care planning, and follows up by monitoring the achievement of desired client outcomes within established time parameters.
- A case manager can be a nurse, social worker, or other designated health care professional. A case manager's role and knowledge expectations are extensive. Therefore, case managers are required to have advanced practice degrees or advanced training in this area.
- Case manager nurses do not usually provide direct client care.
- Case managers usually oversee a caseload of clients who have similar disorders or treatment regimens.
- Case managers in the community coordinate resources and services for clients whose care is based in a residential setting.

NURSING ROLE IN CASE MANAGEMENT

- Coordinating care, particularly for clients who have complex health care needs
- Facilitating continuity of care
- Improving efficiency of care and utilization of resources
- Enhancing quality of care provided
- Limiting unnecessary costs and lengthy stays
- Advocating for the client and family

CRITICAL PATHWAYS

A critical or clinical pathway or care map can be used to support the implementation of clinical guidelines and protocols. These tools are usually based on cost and length of stay parameters mandated by prospective payment systems (Medicare and insurance companies).

- Case managers often initiate critical pathways, but they are used by many members of the interprofessional team.
- Critical pathways are often specific to a diagnosis type and outline the typical length of stay and treatments.
- When a client requires treatment other than what is typical or requires a longer length of stay, it is documented as a variance, along with information describing why the variance occurred.

CONTINUITY OF CARE: CONSULTATIONS, REFERRALS, TRANSFERS, AND DISCHARGE PLANNING

Continuity of care refers to the consistency of care provided as clients move through the health care system. It enhances the quality of client care and facilitates the achievement of positive client outcomes. Q̇PCC

- Continuity of care is desired as clients move from one:
  - Level of care to another (from the ICU to a medical unit).
  - Facility to another (from an acute care facility to a skilled facility).
  - Unit/department to another (from the PACU to the postsurgical unit).
- Nurses are responsible for facilitating continuity of care and coordinating care through documentation, reporting, and collaboration.
- A formal, written plan of care enhances coordination of care between nurses, interprofessional team members, and providers.

NURSING ROLE IN CONTINUITY OF CARE

The nurse's role as coordinator of care includes:
- Facilitating the continuity of care provided by members of the health care team.
- Acting as a representative of the client and as a liaison when collaborating with the provider and other members of the health care team. When acting as a liaison, the nurse serves in the role of client advocate by protecting the rights of clients and ensuring that client needs are met.

As the coordinator of care, the nurse is responsible for:
- Admission, transfer, discharge, and postdischarge prescriptions.
- Initiation, revision, and evaluation of the plan of care.
- Reporting the client's status to other nurses and the provider.
- Coordinating the discharge plan.
- Facilitating referrals and the use of community resources.

DOCUMENTATION

Documentation to facilitate continuity of care includes the following.
- Graphic records that illustrate trending of assessment data (vital signs)
- Flow sheets that reflect routine care completed and other care-related data
- Nurses' notes that describe changes in client status or unusual circumstances
- Client care summaries that serve as quick references for client care information
- Nursing care plans that set the standard for care provided
  - Standardized nursing care plans provide a starting point for the nurse responsible for care plan development.
  - Standardized plans must be individualized to each client.
  - All documentation should reflect the plan of care.

COMMUNICATION AND CONTINUITY OF CARE

- Poor communication can lead to adverse outcomes, including sentinel events (unexpected death or serious injury of a client).
- Communication regarding the client status and needs is required anytime there is a transfer of care, whether from one unit or facility to another, or at change-of-shift, as the nurse hands off the care of the client to another health care professional.
- The guidelines on transfer reporting contain details on what to communicate when transferring client care.

Communication tools
- A number of communication hand-off tools are available to improve communication and promote client safety (I-SBAR, PACE, I PASS the BATON, Five P's). Qs
- Nurses might also communicate interprofessionally through electronic means (through electronic medical record systems and e-mail). Qɪ
  - E-mail communication can be informal, but should maintain a professional tone. Don't use text abbreviations. Make the message concise yet thorough so the reader has clear understanding of the intent.
  - Read messages before sending to ensure there is not a negative or rude tone.
- Some facilities permit text messaging. Check the facility policy regarding this type of communication, and never send confidential information through text.

Hand-off or change-of-shift report
- Performed with the nurse who is assuming responsibility for the client's care.
- Describes the current health status of the client.
- Informs the next shift of pertinent client care information.
- Provides the oncoming nurse the opportunity to ask questions and clarify the plan of care.
- Should be given in a private area (a conference room or at the bedside) to protect client confidentiality.

Report to the provider Qᴛᴄ
- Assessment data integral to changes in client status
- Recommendations for changes in the plan of care
- Clarification of prescriptions

CONSULTATIONS

- A consultant is a professional who provides expert advice in a particular area. A consultation is requested to help determine what treatment/services the client requires.
- Consultants provide expertise for clients who require a specific type of knowledge or service (a cardiologist for a client who had a myocardial infarction, a psychiatrist for a client whose risk for suicide must be assessed).

The nurse's role regarding consultations
- Initiate necessary consults or notify the provider of the client's needs so the consult can be initiated.
- Provide the consultant with all pertinent information about the problem (information from the client/family, the client's medical records).
- Incorporate the consultant's recommendations into the client's plan of care.

REFERRALS

A referral is a formal request for a service by another care provider. It is made so that the client can access the care identified by the provider or the consultant. Qᴘᴄᴄ
- The care can be provided in the acute setting or outside the facility.
- Clients being discharged from health care facilities to their home can still require nursing care.
- Discharge referrals are based on client needs in relation to actual and potential problems and can be facilitated with the assistance of social services, especially if there is a need for:
  - Specialized equipment (cane, walker, wheelchair, grab bars in bathroom)
  - Specialized therapists (physical, occupational, speech)
  - Care providers (home health nurse, hospice nurse, home health aide)
- Knowledge of community and online resources is necessary to appropriately link the client with needed services.

The nurse's role regarding referrals
- Begin discharge planning upon the client's admission.
- Evaluate client/family competencies in relation to home care prior to discharge.
- Involve the client and family in care planning.
- Collaborate with other health care professionals to ensure all health care needs are met and necessary referrals are made.
- Complete referral forms to ensure proper reimbursement for prescribed services.

TRANSFERS

Clients can be transferred from one unit, department, or one facility to another. Continuity of care must be maintained as the client moves from one setting to another.
- The use of communication hand-off tools (I PASS the BATON, PACE) promotes continuity of care and client safety. Qs
- The nurse's role regarding transfers is to provide written and verbal report of the client's status and care needs.
  - Client medical diagnosis and care providers
  - Client demographic information
  - Overview of health status, plan of care, and recent progress
  - Alterations that can precipitate an immediate concern
  - Most recent vital signs and medications, including when a PRN was given
  - Notification of assessments or client care needed within the next few hours
  - Allergies
  - Diet and activity prescriptions
  - Presence of or need for specific equipment or adaptive devices (oxygen, suction, wheelchair)
  - Advance directives and whether a client is to be resuscitated in the event of cardiac or respiratory arrest
  - Family involvement in care and health care proxy, if applicable

DISCHARGE PLANNING

Discharge planning is an interprofessional process that is started by the nurse at the time of the client's admission. Qтс

- The nurse conducts discharge planning with both the client and client's family for optimal results.
- Discharge planning serves as a starting point for continuity of care. As client care needs are identified, measures can be taken to prepare for the provision of needed support.
- A comprehensive discharge plan includes a review of the following client information.
  - Current health and prognosis
  - Religious or cultural beliefs
  - Ability to perform ADLs
  - Mobility status and goals
  - Sensory, motor, physical, or cognitive impairments
  - Support systems and caregivers
  - Financial resources and limitations
  - Potential supports and resources in the community
  - Internal and external home environment
  - Need for assistance with transportation or home maintenance
  - Need for therapy, wound care, or other services
  - Need for medical equipment
- The need for additional services (home health, physical therapy, and respite care) can be addressed before the client is discharged so the service is in place when the client arrives home.
- A client who leaves a facility without a prescription for discharge from the provider is considered leaving against medical advice (AMA). A client who is legally competent has the legal right to leave the facility at any time. The nurse should immediately notify the provider. If the client is at risk for harm, it is imperative that the nurse explain the risk involved in leaving the facility. The individual should sign a form relinquishing responsibility for any complications that arise from discontinuing prescribed care. The nurse should document all communication, as well as the specific advice that was provided for the client. A nurse who tries to prevent the client from leaving the facility can face legal charges of assault, battery, and false imprisonment.

Discharge instructions

- Step-by-step instructions for procedures to be done at home. Clients should be given the opportunity to provide a return demonstration of these procedures to validate learning.
- Medication regimen instructions for home, including adverse effects and actions to take to minimize them.
- Precautions to take when performing procedures or administering medications.
- Indications of medication adverse effects or medical complications that the client should report to the provider.
- Names and numbers of providers and community services the client or family can contact.
- Plans for follow-up care and therapies.

The nurse's role with regard to discharge is to provide a written summary including:

- Type of discharge (prescribed by provider, AMA).
- Date and time of discharge, who accompanied the client, and how the client was transported (wheelchair to a private car, stretcher to an ambulance).
- Discharge destination (home, long-term care facility).
- A summary of the client's condition at discharge (gait, dietary intake, use of assistive devices, blood glucose).
- A description of any unresolved problems and plans for follow-up.
- Disposition of valuables, medications brought from home, and prescriptions.
- A copy of the client's discharge instructions.

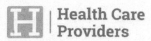 **Health Care Providers**

INTERFACILITY TRANSER FORM

1234 Main Street
Shermer, IL 12345
1.800.555.1234

TRANSFER FROM: _____

Client condition: ☐ Stable ☐ Unstable

Reason for transfer and Benefits and Risks of transfer:
☐ Client/responsible person's request
☐ Need for higher level of care not available at this facility
☐ Need for diagnostic equipment not available at this facility
☐ Transfer request by:
☐ Other: _____

Benefits of Transfer: _____

_____

Risks of Transfer:
☐ Death
☐ Vehicular accident
☐ Bleeding
☐ Pulmonary Decompensation
☐ Cardiac Decompensation
☐ Delivery in route
☐ Deterioration of medical condition:
☐ Additional delay in receiving appropriate treatment
☐ Other

_____ I certify that based upon the information available at the time of transfer, the medical benefits and treatment at the accepting facility, outweigh the increased risks to the client in the case of pregnancy, the unborn infant.

_____ After client assessment, I certify that I have discussed the risks and benefits to the client that were known to me at the time of transfer.

Medical Diagnosis: _____

_____

Provider's Name: _____
Signature: _____
Date: _____ Time: _____

I acknowledge by my signature that I agree to my transfer to the receiving facility and the transferring provider has discussed with me the risks and benefits of transfer.

Client Signature: _____
Client unable to sign, signature
of responsible person: _____
Relationship: _____

Approval of Transfer

_____ The receiving facility has agreed to accept the client, provide appropriate medical treatment and has available and qualified personnel for the treatment of this client.

Name/title of transferring facility
contact receiving above approval: _____
Name/title of receiving facility
contact granting above approval: _____
Name of receiving facility: _____
Name of provider receiving client
from transferring provider: _____
Name of transferring nursing
personnel giving report: _____
Name of receiving nursing
personnel receiving report: _____
Available space confirmed by: _____
Time: _____

Method of Transfer

Name of transferring facility: _____
Time of arrival: _____ Time of transfer: _____
Qualified personnel with appropriate medical equipment which will be able to use all necessary and appropriate life support measures will transfer the client:
☐ BLS ☐ ALS ☐ Air transport ☐ Other: _____

Treatment

_____ The transferring facility has within its capacity provided medical treatment to minimize the risk to the client's health (and in the case of pregnancy, the unborn infant).

Treatment rendered included:
☐ IV:
☐ Medications:
☐ Oxygen:
☐ Procedures:

Vital signs at the time of transfer:
T_____ P_____ R_____ BP_____

Records sent with client:
☐ Laboratory findings:
☐ Radiographs:
☐ EKG   Valuables
☐ Medical record   ☐ To the family
Discharge client assessment: _____

Name of Transferring Nurse: _____
Signature: _____ Date: _____

H | Health Care Providers

TRANSFER REPORT

1234 Main Street
Shermer, IL 12345
1.800.555.1234

Name: _____ DOB: _____

Admission date: _____ Medical record #: _____

Transfer date: _____ Attending provider: _____

Transfer from: _____ Address: _____

Transfer to: _____ Phone: _____

Contact: _____ Notify ☐ Yes ☐ No

Address: _____

Phone: _____

Relationship: _____

Reason for transfer

Vital signs:

T _____ P _____ R _____ BP _____ WT _____

Diagnosis: _____

Prognosis/rehab potential: _____

Allergies: _____

Diet: _____

Activity level: _____

Precautions: _____

ADLs

	No assistance needed	Assistance/ supervision	Total care
Walking			
Transfers			
Bathing			
Eating			
Oral hygiene			
Dressing			

Medication:	Date/time of last dose:
Treatment:	Date/time:

Prosthesis: _____

Hearing: _____

Speech: _____

Vision: _____

Bowel/bladder: _____

Mental status: _____

Emotional status: _____

Additional information: _____

Provider signature: _____ Nurse signature: _____

Date: _____ Date: _____

Patient Discharge Summary

H **Health Care Providers**
1234 Main Street
Shermer, IL 12345
1.800.555.1234

Name: _____   SSN: _____
Address: _____   DOB: _____
Email address: _____   Sex: ☐ Male ☐ Female

Reason for admittance: _____

Diagnosis at admittance: _____

Treatment summary: _____
_____
_____
_____
_____

Discharge reason: Discharge state: Date discharged: _____
☐ Needs met   ☐ Independent   Physician approved: ☐ Yes   ☐ No
☐ Patient deceased   ☐ Assistance required: minimal   Diagnosis at discharge: _____
☐ Hospital admission   ☐ Assistance required: moderate   _____
☐ Moved away   ☐ Assistance required: maximal   Further treatment plan: _____
☐ Refused services   ☐ Assistance required: total   _____
☐ Discharge to outpatient therapy   _____
☐ Transferred: hospice services   _____
☐ Transferred: other home health services   Follow up with provider? ☐ Yes   ☐ No
☐ Transferred: nursing home   Follow-up date: _____

Notes: _____
_____
_____
_____
_____

Medication information:
(include name, dose and route)   *Frequency*   *Instructions/adverse effects*
_____   _____   _____
_____   _____   _____
_____   _____   _____
_____   _____   _____
_____   _____   _____
_____   _____   _____
_____   _____   _____

                                                            Signature: _____
                                                            Date: _____

1. A nurse is preparing to transfer a client who is 72 hr postoperative to a long-term care facility. Which of the following information should the nurse include in the transfer report? (Select all that apply).

   A. Type of anesthesia used

   B. Advance directives status

   C. Vital signs on day of admission

   D. Medical diagnosis

   E. Need for specific equipment

2. A nurse is assisting with the discharge planning for a client. Which of the following actions should the nurse take? (Select all that apply.)

   A. Determine the client's need for home medical equipment.

   B. Provide a list of all the medications the client received in the facility.

   C. Obtain printed instructions for medication self-administration.

   D. Provide the family with a list of community agencies that can provide assistance.

   E. Discuss the importance of attending follow-up appointments.

3. A case manager is discussing critical pathways with a group of newly hired nurses. Which of the following statements indicates understanding?

   A. "The time to fill out the pathways often increases the cost of care."

   B. "The pathway shows an estimate of the number of days the client will be hospitalized."

   C. "Deviance from the pathway is a sign of improved care quality."

   D. "The pathway includes information about the client's history."

4. A nurse who has just assumed the role of unit manager is examining the skills necessary for interprofessional collaboration. Which of the following actions support the nurse's interprofessional collaboration? (Select all that apply.)

   A. Use aggressive communication when addressing the team.

   B. Recognize the knowledge and skills of each member of the team.

   C. Ensure that a nurse is assigned to serve as the group facilitator for all interprofessional meetings.

   D. Encourage the client and family to participate in the team meeting.

   E. Support team member requests for referral.

5. A nurse is caring for a client who has chest pain. The client says, "I am going home immediately." Which of the following actions should the nurse take? (Select all that apply.)

   A. Notify the client's family of their intent to leave the facility.

   B. Document the client's intent to leave the facility against medical advice (AMA).

   C. Explain to the client the risks involved if they choose to leave.

   D. Ask the client to sign a form relinquishing responsibility of the facility.

   E. Prevent the client from leaving the facility until the provider arrives.

Active Learning Scenario

A nurse is explaining the role of a case manager to a newly licensed nurse. What should the case manager include in the discussion? Use the ATI Active Learning Template: Basic Concept to complete this item.

UNDERLYING PRINCIPLES: Identify three roles of a case manager.

Application Exercises Key

1. A. The receiving nurse and facility do not need to know the type of anesthesia used in order to provide care or address the client's current needs.
   B. **CORRECT:** Communicate the client's advance directive status as part of client advocacy.
   C. The receiving nurse and facility do not need to know admission vital signs in order to provide care or address the client's current needs. However, provide the most recent set of vital signs in the report.
   D. **CORRECT:** Communicate the client's medical diagnosis in order to provide care and address the client's current needs.
   E. **CORRECT:** Communicate the client's need for specific equipment so the facility can provide appropriate care.

   Ⓝ *NCLEX® Connection: Management of Care, Continuity of Care*

2. A. **CORRECT:** Determine whether the client will need home medical equipment so that the process of acquiring the equipment can begin.
   B. Provide the client a list of currently prescribed medications so that the client can continue to take the correct medications at home.
   C. **CORRECT:** Provide instructions about medications and procedures to perform at home.
   D. **CORRECT:** Inform the client and family about community agencies that can help provide resources or assist with client care.
   E. **CORRECT:** Ensure the client has follow-up appointments scheduled and knows when to contact the provider otherwise to prevent or minimize health complications.

   Ⓝ *NCLEX® Connection: Management of Care, Collaboration with Interdisciplinary Team*

3. A. Critical pathways often reduce the cost of care by streamlining care services.
   B. **CORRECT:** Critical pathways are specific to a client diagnosis and show the average length of stay a client with the diagnosis type will have.
   C. Deviances from the pathway require documentation of explanation, because it usually indicates the client is not progressing at the expected rate.
   D. Critical pathways include a projection of treatments the client will receive.

   Ⓝ *NCLEX® Connection: Management of Care, Concepts of Management*

4. A. The nurse should use assertive skills when communicating with the interprofessional team.
   B. **CORRECT:** The nurse should recognize that each member of the team has specific skills to contribute to the collaboration process.
   C. A nurse can serve as the facilitator. However, this role can be assumed by any member of the team.
   D. **CORRECT:** Collaboration should occur among the client, family, and interprofessional team.
   E. **CORRECT:** The nurse should support suggestions for referrals to link clients to appropriate resources.

   Ⓝ *NCLEX® Connection: Management of Care, Collaboration with Interdisciplinary Team*

5. A. Notifying the client's family without the client's permission violates the client's right to confidentiality. Notify the client's provider.
   B. **CORRECT:** When documenting a discharge, document the type of discharge, including an AMA discharge.
   C. **CORRECT:** The nurse is legally responsible to warn the client of the risks involved in leaving the hospital against medical advice.
   D. **CORRECT:** Clients who leave the hospital prior to a prescribed discharge are asked to sign a form to provide legal protection for the hospital.
   E. A nurse who tries to prevent a client from leaving the hospital by any action (threatening them or refusing to give them their clothes) can be charged with assault, battery, and false imprisonment.

   Ⓝ *NCLEX® Connection: Management of Care, Client Rights*

Active Learning Scenario Key

Using the ATI Active Learning Template: Basic Concept

UNDERLYING PRINCIPLES: Roles of a case manager
- Coordinating care of clients who have complex health care needs
- Facilitating continuity of care
- Improving efficiency of care
- Enhancing quality of care provided
- Limiting cost and lengthy stays
- Advocating for the client and family

Ⓝ *NCLEX® Connection: Management of Care, Concepts of Management*

When reviewing the following chapter, keep in mind the relevant topics and tasks of the NCLEX outline, in particular:

Management of Care

ADVANCE DIRECTIVES/SELF-DETERMINATION/LIFE PLANNING: Integrate advance directives into client plan of care.

ADVOCACY: Discuss identified treatment options with client and respect their decisions.

CLIENT RIGHTS: Provide education to clients and staff about client rights and responsibilities.

CONFIDENTIALITY/INFORMATION SECURITY: Assess staff member and client understanding of confidentiality requirements.

ETHICAL PRACTICE: Recognize ethical dilemmas and take appropriate action.

INFORMED CONSENT: Verify the client receives appropriate education and consents to care and procedures.

INFORMATION TECHNOLOGY: Apply knowledge of facility regulations when accessing client records.

LEGAL RIGHTS AND RESPONSIBILITIES: Educate the client/staff on legal issues.

Safety and Infection Control

REPORTING OF INCIDENT/EVENT/IRREGULAR OCCURRENCE/VARIANCE: Report unsafe practice of health care personnel and intervene as appropriate (e.g., substance abuse, improper care, staffing practices).

CHAPTER 3 *Professional Responsibilities*

Professional responsibilities are the obligations that nurses have to their clients. To meet their professional responsibilities, nurses must be knowledgeable in the following areas: client rights, advocacy, informed consent, advance directives, confidentiality and information security, information technology, legal practice, disruptive behavior, and ethical practice.

Client rights

- Client rights are the legal guarantees that clients have with regard to their health care.
  - Clients using the services of a health care institution retain their rights as individuals and citizens of the United States. The American Hospital Association (AHA) identifies client rights in health care settings in the Patient Care Partnership (www.aha.org).
  - Residents in nursing facilities that participate in Medicare programs similarly retain resident rights under statutes that govern the operation of these facilities.
- Nurses are accountable for protecting the rights of clients. Situations that require particular attention include informed consent, refusal of treatment, advance directives, confidentiality, and information security.

NURSING ROLE IN CLIENT RIGHTS

- Nurses must ensure that clients understand their rights. Nurses also must protect clients' rights during nursing care. Q**PCC**
- Regardless of the client's age, nursing needs, or the setting in which care is provided, the basic tenants are the same. Each client has the right to the following.
  - Be informed about all aspects of care and take an active role in the decision-making process.
  - Accept, refuse, or request modification to the plan of care.
  - Receive care that is delivered by competent individuals who treat the client with respect.

REFUSAL OF TREATMENT

The Patient Self-Determination Act (PSDA) stipulates that on admission to a health care facility, all clients must be informed of their right to accept or refuse care. Competent adults have the right to refuse treatment, including the right to leave a health care facility without a prescription for discharge from the provider.

- If the client refuses a treatment or procedure, the client is asked to sign a document indicating that they understand the risk involved with refusing the treatment or procedure, and that they have chosen to refuse it.
- When a client decides to leave the facility without a prescription for discharge, the nurse notifies the provider and discusses with the client the potential risks associated with leaving the facility prior to discharge.
- The nurse carefully documents the information that was provided to the client and that notification of the provider occurred. The client should be informed of the following.
  - Possible complications that could occur without treatment
  - Possibility of permanent physical or mental impairment or disability
  - Possibility of other complications that could lead to death
- The client is asked to sign an Against Medical Advice form.
- If the client refuses to sign the form, this is also documented by the nurse.

Advocacy

Advocacy refers to nurses' role in supporting clients by ensuring that they are properly informed, that their rights are respected, and that they are receiving the proper level of care.

- Advocacy is one of the most important roles of the nurse, especially when clients are unable to speak or act for themselves.
- As an advocate, the nurse ensures that the client has the information they need to make decisions about health care.
- Nurses must act as advocates even when they disagree with clients' decisions.
- The complex health care system puts clients in a vulnerable position. Nurses are clients' voice when the system is not acting in their best interest.
- The nursing profession also has a responsibility to support and advocate for legislation that promotes public policies that protect clients as consumers and create a safe environment for their care.

NURSING ROLE IN ADVOCACY

- As advocates, nurses must ensure that clients are informed of their rights and have adequate information on which to base health care decisions.
- Nurses must be careful to assist clients with making health care decisions and not direct or control their decisions.
- Nurses mediate on the client's behalf when the actions of others are not in the client's best interest or changes need to be made in the plan of care.
- Situations in which nurses might need to advocate for clients or assist them to advocate for themselves include the following.
  ○ End-of-life decisions
  ○ Access to health care
  ○ Protection of client privacy
  ○ Informed consent
  ○ Substandard practice
- Nurses are accountable for their actions even if they are carrying out a provider's prescription. It is the nurse's responsibility to question a prescription if it could harm a client (incorrect medication dosage, potential adverse interaction with another prescribed medication, contraindication due to an allergy or medical history). Qs

ESSENTIAL COMPONENTS OF ADVOCACY

SKILLS

- Risk-taking
- Vision
- Self-confidence
- Articulate communication
- Assertiveness

VALUES

- Caring
- Autonomy
- Respect
- Empowerment

Informed consent

- Informed consent is a legal process by which a client has given written permission for a procedure or treatment to be performed. Consent is considered to be informed when the client has been provided with and understands the following.
  ○ Reason the treatment or procedure is needed
  ○ How the treatment or procedure will benefit the client
  ○ Risks involved if the client chooses to receive the treatment or procedure
  ○ Other options to treat the problem, including the option of not treating the problem
  ○ Risk involved if the client chooses no treatment
- The nurse's role in the informed consent process is to witness the client's signature on the informed consent form and to ensure that informed consent has been appropriately obtained.
- The nurse should seek the assistance of an interpreter if the client does not speak and understand the language used by the provider. Qpcc

INFORMED CONSENT GUIDELINES

Consent is required for all care given in a health care facility. For most aspects of nursing care, implied consent is adequate. The client provides implied consent when they comply with the instructions provided by the nurse. For example, the nurse is preparing to administer a TB skin test, and the client holds out their arm for the nurse.

- For an invasive procedure or surgery, the client is required to provide written consent.
- State laws regulate who is able to give informed consent. Laws vary regarding age limitations and emergencies. Nurses are responsible for knowing the laws in the state of practice.
- The nurse must verify that consent is informed and witness the client sign the consent form.

Signing an informed consent form

- The form for informed consent must be signed by a competent adult.
  ○ Emancipated minors (minors who are independent from their parents [a married minor]) can provide informed consent for themselves.
- The person who signs the form must be capable of understanding the information provided by the health care professional who will be providing the service. The person must be able to fully communicate in return with the health care professional.
- When the person giving the informed consent is unable to communicate due to a language barrier or hearing impairment, a trained medical interpreter must be provided. Many health care agencies contract with professional interpreters who have additional skills in medical terminology to assist with providing information.

Individuals authorized to grant consent for another person

- Parent of a minor
- Legal guardian
- Court-specified representative
- Client's health care surrogate (individual who has the client's durable power of attorney for health care/health care proxy)
- Spouse or closest available relative (state laws vary)

INFORMED CONSENT RESPONSIBILITIES

PROVIDER: Obtains informed consent. To do so, the provider must give the client the following.

- Complete description of the treatment/procedure
- Description of the professionals who will be performing and participating in the treatment
- Description of the potential harm, pain, and/or discomfort that might occur
- Options for other treatments and the possible consequences of taking other actions
- The right to refuse treatment
- Risk involved if the client chooses no treatment

CLIENT: Gives informed consent. To give informed consent, the client must do the following.

- Give it voluntarily (no coercion involved).
- Be competent and of legal age, or be an emancipated minor. (If the client is unable to provide consent, an authorized person must give consent.)
- Receive sufficient information to make a decision based on an informed understanding of what is expected.

NURSE

- Witnesses informed consent. The nurse is responsible for the following. **Qs**
  - Ensuring that the provider gave the client the necessary information
  - Ensuring that the client understood the information and is competent to give informed consent
  - Having the client sign the informed consent document
  - Notifying the provider if the client has more questions or does not understand any of the information provided (The provider is then responsible for giving clarification.)
- The nurse documents the following.
  - Reinforcement of information originally given by the provider
  - That questions the client had were forwarded to the provider
  - Use of an interpreter

Advance directives

- The purpose of advance directives is to communicate a client's wishes regarding end-of-life care should the client become unable to do so.
- The PSDA requires that all clients admitted to a health care facility be asked if they have advance directives.
  - A client who does not have advance directives must be given written information that outlines their rights related to health care decisions and how to formulate advance directives. **Qpcc**
  - A health care representative should be available to help with this process.

COMPONENTS OF ADVANCE DIRECTIVES

Two components of an advance directive are the living will and the durable power of attorney for health care.

Living will

- A living will is a legal document that expresses the client's wishes regarding medical treatment in the event the client becomes incapacitated and is facing end-of-life issues. Types of treatments that are often addressed in a living will are those that have the capacity to prolong life. Examples of treatments that are addressed are cardiopulmonary resuscitation, mechanical ventilation, and feeding by artificial means.
- Living wills are legal in all states. However, state statutes and individual health care facility policies can vary. Nurses need to be familiar with their state statute and facility policies.
- Most state laws include provisions that health care providers who follow the health care directive in a living will are protected from liability.

Durable power of attorney for health care

A durable power of attorney for health care/health care proxy is a legal document that designates a health care surrogate, who is an individual authorized to make health care decisions for a client who is unable.

- The person who serves in the role of health care surrogate to make decisions for the client should be very familiar with the client's wishes.
- Living wills can be difficult to interpret, especially in the face of unexpected circumstances. A durable power of attorney for health care, as an adjunct to a living will, can be a more effective way of ensuring that the client's decisions about health care are honored.

Provider's prescriptions

- Unless a do not resuscitate (DNR) or allow natural death (AND) prescription is written, the nurse should initiate CPR when a client has no pulse or respirations. The written prescription for a DNR or AND must be placed in the client's medical record. The provider consults the client and the family prior to administering a DNR or AND.
- Additional prescriptions by the provider are based on the client's individual needs and decisions and provide for comfort measures. The client's decision is respected in regard to the use of antibiotics, initiation of diagnostic tests, and provision of nutrition by artificial means.

NURSING ROLE IN ADVANCE DIRECTIVES

- Providing written information regarding advance directives
- Documenting the client's advance directives status
- Ensuring that advance directives are current and reflective of the client's current decisions
- Recognizing that the client's choice takes priority when there is a conflict between the client and family, or between the client and the provider
- Informing all members of the health care team of the client's advance directives Qpcc

Confidentiality and information security

Clients have the right to privacy and confidentiality in relation to their health care information and medical recommendations.

- Nurses who disclose client information to an unauthorized person can be liable for invasion of privacy, defamation, or slander.
- The security and privacy rules of the Health Insurance Portability and Accountability Act (HIPAA) were enacted to protect the confidentiality of health care information and to give the client the right to control the release of information. Specific rights provided by the legislation include the following:
  - The rights of clients to obtain a copy of their medical record and to submit requests to amend erroneous or incomplete information
  - A requirement for health care and insurance providers to provide written information about how medical information is used and how it is shared with other entities (permission must be obtained before information is shared)
  - The rights of clients to privacy and confidentiality

NURSING ROLE IN CONFIDENTIALITY

It is essential for nurses to be aware of the rights of clients in regard to privacy and confidentiality. Facility policies and procedures are established in order to ensure compliance with HIPAA regulations. It is essential that nurses know and adhere to the policies and procedures. HIPAA regulations also provide for penalties in the event of noncompliance with the regulations. Qs

PRIVACY RULE

The Privacy Rule of HIPAA requires that nurses protect all written and verbal communication about clients.

COMPONENTS OF THE PRIVACY RULE
- Only health care team members directly responsible for the client's care are allowed access to the client's records. Nurses cannot share information with other clients or staff not involved in the care of the client.
- Clients have a right to read and obtain a copy of their medical record, and agency policy should be followed when the client requests to read or have a copy of the record.
- No part of the client record can be copied except for authorized exchange of documents between health care institutions. For example:
  - Transfer from a hospital to an extended care facility
  - Exchange of documents between a general practitioner and a specialist during a consult
- Client medical records must be kept in a secure area to prevent inappropriate access to the information. Using public display boards to list client names and diagnoses is restricted.
- Electronic records should be password-protected, and care must be taken to prevent public viewing of the information. Health care workers should use only their own passwords to access information.
- Client information cannot be disclosed to unauthorized individuals, including family members who request it and individuals who call on the phone.
  - Many hospitals use a code system in which information is only disclosed to individuals who can provide the code.
  - Nurses should ask any individual inquiring about a client's status for the code and disclose information only when an individual can give the code.
- Communication about a client should only take place in a private setting where it cannot be overheard by unauthorized individuals. The practice of "walking rounds," where other clients and visitors can hear what is being said, is no longer sanctioned. Taped rounds also are discouraged because nurses should not receive information about clients for whom they are not responsible. Change-of-shift reports can be done at the bedside as long as the client does not have a roommate and no unsolicited visitors are present. Qpcc

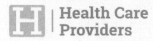 **Health Care Providers**

ADVANCE DIRECTIVE
Living Will/Power of Attorney for Health Care

1234 Main Street
Shermer, IL 12345
1.800.555.1234

On this _____ day of _____, I, _____, being of sound mind, willfully designate the following individual, _____, as my agent to make all health care related decisions for me.

If, for any reason, should I revoke my agent's authority or if my agent is not willing, able, or available to make health care decisions for me, I designate as my first alternate, _____.

MY AGENT shall have the authority to make health care decisions that will become effective if and when my primary physician determines that I am unable, either physically and/or mentally, to make my own decisions regarding my health care.

MY AGENT shall have the authority to make health care decisions in what he/she determines is my best interest and carry out any instructions that I mark as my own will to be done.

MY AGENT shall be in accordance with my following choice:

☐ Choice NOT to Prolong Life
   I do not want to be resuscitated in the event I (1) have an incurable and irreversible condition that will result in my death within a short period of time, (2) become unconscious and have little or no chance of regaining consciousness, or (3) the risks of treatment would outweigh the expected benefits.

☐ Choice To Prolong Life
   I want my life to be prolonged as long as possible within the scope and limits of accepted health care standards.

MY AGENT shall direct that treatment for alleviation of pain or discomfort should be provided at all times even if it directly affects the demise of my health or hastens my death.

MY AGENT shall donate my organs as specified below.

☐ I give all organs, tissues, or parts
☐ I give the following organs, tissues, or parts ONLY:
☐ My gift is for the following purposes (Place a mark in the box next to the desired purpose(s) for donation):
   ☐ Transplant
   ☐ Therapy
   ☐ Research
   ☐ Education

MY AGENT shall, upon my death, make health care decisions regarding authorization of an autopsy, making anatomical gifts, and the disposition of my remains.

This Power of Attorney will not be effective unless it is signed by me, my designated agent, my alternative agent and my primary physician.

Signature: _____ Date: _____

Signature: _____ Date: _____

Signature: _____ Date: _____

Physician Signature: _____ Date: _____

INFORMATION SECURITY

- Health information systems (HIS) are used to manage administrative functions and clinical functions. The clinical portion of the system is often referred to as the clinical information systems (CIS). The CIS can be used to coordinate essential aspects of client care. Q↓
- In order to comply with HIPAA regulations, each health care facility has specific policies and procedures designed to monitor staff adherence, technical protocols, computer privacy, and data safety.

INFORMATION SECURITY PROTOCOLS

- Log off from the computer before leaving the workstation to ensure that others cannot view protected health information (PHI) on the monitor.
- Never share a user ID or password with anyone.
- Never leave a client's chart or other printed or written PHI where others can access it.
- Shred any printed or written client information used for reporting or client care after it is no longer needed.

USE OF SOCIAL MEDIA

- The use of social media by members of the nursing profession is common practice. The benefits to using social media are numerous. It provides a mechanism for nurses to access current information about health care and enhances communication among nurses, colleagues, and clients and families. It also provides an opportunity for nurses to express concerns and seek support from others. However, nurses must be cautious about the risk of intentional or inadvertent breaches of confidentiality via social media.
- The right to privacy is a fundamental component of client care. Invasion of privacy as it relates to health care is the release of client health information to others without the client's consent. Confidentiality is the duty of the nurse to protect a client's private information.
- The inappropriate use of social media can result in a breach of client confidentiality. Depending on the circumstances, the consequences can include termination of employment by the employer, discipline by the board of nursing, charges of defamation or invasion of privacy, and in the most serious of circumstances, federal charges for violation of HIPAA.

Protecting yourself and others

- Become familiar with facility policies about the use of social media, and adhere to them.
- Avoid disclosing any client health information online. Be sure no one can overhear conversations about a client when speaking on the telephone.
- Do not take or share photos or videos of a client.
- Remember to maintain professional boundaries when interacting with clients online.
- Never post a belittling or offensive remark about a client, employer, or coworker.
- Report any violations of facility social media policies to the nurse manager.

Information technology

- Informatics is the use of computers to systematically resolve issues in nursing. The use of technology in health care is increasing and most forms of communication are in electronic format. Q↓
- Examples of how a nurse can use the electronic format while providing client care include laptops for documentation and the use of an automated medication dispensing system to dispense medications.
- Databases on diseases and medications are available for the nurse to review. These databases can also be used as a teaching tool when nurses are educating clients.
- The nurse can review medications, diseases, procedures, and treatments using an electronic format.
- Computers can be beneficial for use with clients who have visual impairments.
- The Internet is a valuable tool for clients to review current medications and health questions. This is especially true for clients who have chronic illnesses.
- Nurses should instruct clients to only review valid and credible websites by verifying the author, institution, credentials, and how current the article is. A disclaimer will be presented if information is not medical advice.
- Clients can access their electronic health record (EHR) which is part of e-health. E-health enables the client to make appointments online, review laboratory results, refill an electronic prescription, and review billing information. The goal of e-health is improved health care outcomes due to 24 hr access by the client and provider to the client's health care information.

Legal practice

In order to be safe practitioners, nurses must understand the legal aspects of the nursing profession. Qs

- Understanding the laws governing nursing practice allows nurses to protect client rights and reduce the risk of nursing liability.
- Nurses are accountable for practicing nursing in accordance with the various sources of law affecting nursing practice. It is important that nurses know and comply with these laws. By practicing nursing within the confines of the law, nurses are able to do the following.
  - Provide safe, competent care
  - Advocate for clients' rights
  - Provide care that is within the nurse's scope of practice
  - Discern the responsibilities of nursing in relation to the responsibilities of other members of the health care team
  - Provide care that is consistent with established standards of care
  - Shield oneself from liability

SOURCES OF LAW

Federal regulations

Federal regulations have a great impact on nursing practice. Some of the federal laws affecting nursing practice include the following.
- HIPAA
- Americans with Disabilities Act (ADA)
- Mental Health Parity Act (MHPA)
- Patient Self-Determination Act (PSDA)
- Uniform Anatomical Gift Act (UAGA)
- National Organ Transplant Act (NOTA)
- Emergency Medical Treatment and Active Labor Act (EMTALA)

Criminal and civil laws

Criminal law is a subsection of public law and relates to the relationship of an individual with the government. Violations of criminal law can be categorized as either a **felony** (a serious crime [homicide]) or **misdemeanor** (a less serious crime [petty theft]). A nurse who falsifies a record to cover up a serious mistake can be found guilty of breaking a criminal law.

Civil laws protect the individual rights of people. One type of civil law that relates to the provision of nursing care is tort law. Torts can be classified as unintentional, quasi-intentional, or intentional.

Unintentional torts
- **Negligence:** Practice or misconduct that does not meet expected standards of care and places the client at risk for injury (a nurse fails to implement safety measures for a client who has been identified as at risk for falls).
- **Malpractice:** Professional negligence (a nurse administers a large dose of medication due to a calculation error. The client has a cardiac arrest and dies).

Quasi-intentional torts
- **Invasion of privacy:** Intrusion into a client's private affairs or a breach of confidentiality (a nurse releases the medical diagnosis of a client to a member of the press).
- **Defamation:** False communication or communication with careless disregard for the truth with the intent to injure an individual's reputation.
  - **Libel:** Defamation with the written word or photographs (a nurse documents in a client's health record that a provider is incompetent).
  - **Slander:** Defamation with the spoken word (a nurse tells a coworker that she believes a client has been unfaithful to the spouse).

Intentional torts
- **Assault:** The conduct of one person makes another person fearful and apprehensive (threatening to place a nasogastric tube in a client who is refusing to eat).
- **Battery:** Intentional and wrongful physical contact with a person that involves an injury or offensive contact (restraining a client and administering an injection against their wishes).
- **False imprisonment:** A competent person not at risk for injury to self or others is confined or restrained against their will (using restraints on a competent client to prevent their leaving the health care facility).

State laws

- The core of nursing practice is regulated by state law.
- Each state has enacted statutes that define the parameters of nursing practice and give the authority to regulate the practice of nursing to its state board of nursing.
  - Boards of nursing have the authority to adopt rules and regulations that further regulate nursing practice. Although the practice of nursing is similar among states, it is critical that nurses know the laws and rules governing nursing in the state in which they practice.
  - The laws and rules governing nursing practice in a specific state can be accessed at the state board's website.
  - Boards of nursing have the authority to both issue and revoke a nursing license. Boards can revoke or suspend a nurse's license for a number of offenses, including practicing without a valid license, substance use disorders, conviction of a felony, professional negligence, and providing care beyond the scope of practice. Nurses should review the practice act in their states.
  - Boards also set standards for nursing programs and further delineate the scope of practice for registered nurses, licensed practical nurses, and advanced practice nurses.
- State laws vary as to when an individual can begin practicing nursing. Some states allow graduates of nursing programs to practice under a limited license, whereas some states require licensure by passing the NCLEX® before working.

Good Samaritan laws

Good Samaritan laws, which vary from state to state, protect nurses who provide emergency assistance outside of the employment location. The nurse must provide a standard of care that is reasonable and prudent.

Licensure

- Until the year 2000, nurses were required to hold a current license in every state in which they practiced. This became problematic with the increase in the electronic practice of nursing. For example, a nurse in one state interprets the reading of a cardiac monitor and provides intervention for a client who is physically located in another state. Additionally, many nurses cross state lines to provide direct care. For example, a nurse who is located near a state border makes home visits on both sides of the state line.
- To address these issues, the mutual recognition model of nurse licensure (the Nurse Licensure Compact [NLC]) has been adopted by many states. This model allows nurses who reside in a NLC state to practice in another NLC state. Nurses must practice in accordance with the statues and rules of the state in which the care is provided. State boards can prohibit a nurse from practicing under the NLC if the license of the nurse has been restricted by a board of nursing.

- Nurses who do not reside in a NLC state must practice under the state-based practice model. In other words, if a nurse resides in a non-NLC state, the nurse must maintain a current license in every state in which they practice. Some states now require background checks with licensure renewal. It is illegal to practice nursing with an expired license.
- The Enhanced Nurse Licensure Compact (eNLC) was revised in 2017. It aligned licensing standards (criminal history background checks) in an effort to bring more states into the compact. Nurses in eNLC states have one multistate license, with the ability to practice in-person or via telehealth in both their home state and other eNLC states.

MALPRACTICE (PROFESSIONAL NEGLIGENCE)

- Malpractice is the failure of a person with professional training to act in a reasonable and prudent manner. The terms "reasonable and prudent" are generally used to describe a person who has the average judgment, foresight, intelligence, and skill that would be expected of a person with similar training and experience. **(3.2)**
- Professional negligence issues that prompt most malpractice suits include failure to do the following.
  - Follow either professional or facility established standards of care
  - Use equipment in a responsible and knowledgeable manner
  - Communicate effectively and thoroughly with the client
  - Document care that was provided
- Nurses can avoid being liable for negligence by doing the following.
  - Following standards of care
  - Giving competent care
  - Communicating with other health team members
  - Developing a caring rapport with clients
  - Fully documenting assessments, interventions, and evaluations

STANDARDS OF CARE (PRACTICE)

- Nurses base practice on established standards of care or legal guidelines for care. These standards of care can be found in the following.
  - The nurse practice act of each state
    - These acts govern nursing practice, and legal guidelines for practice are established and enforced through a state board of nursing or other government agency.
    - Nurse practice acts vary from state to state, making it obligatory for the nurse to be informed about their state's nurse practice act as it defines the legal parameters of practice.
  - Published standards of nursing practice: These are developed by professional organizations (the American Nurses Association, National Association of Practical Nurse Education and Services, Inc.) and specialty organizations (the American Association of Critical Care Nurses; Wound, Ostomy and Continence Nurses Society; and Oncology Nurses Society).
  - Accrediting bodies (The Joint Commission)
  - Originally mandated quality assurance programs, which have evolved into quality improvement
  - Sentinel event reporting: "An unexpected occurrence involving death or serious or psychological injury, or the risk thereof"
  - Failure Mode and Effects Analysis: Examines all potential failures in a design, including event sequencing risks, vulnerabilities, and improvement areas
  - National Patient Safety Goals: Augments core measures and promotes client safety through client identification, effective staff communication, safe medication use, infection prevention, safety risk identification, and preventing wrong-site surgery
  - Health care facility policies and procedures
    - Policies and procedures, maintained in the facility's policy and procedure manual, establish the standard of practice for employees of that institution.
    - These manuals provide detailed information about how the nurse should respond to or provide care in specific situations and while performing client care procedures.
    - Nurses who practice according to institutional policy are legally protected if that standard of care still results in an injury. For example, if a client files a complaint with the board of nursing or seeks legal counsel, the nurse who has followed the facility's policies will not usually be charged with misconduct.
    - It is very important that nurses are familiar with their institution's policies and procedures and provide client care in accordance with these policies. For example:
      - Assess and document findings postoperatively according to institutional policy.
      - Change IV tubing and flush saline locks according to institutional policy.

- Standards of care guide, define, and direct the level of care that should be given by practicing nurses. They also are used in malpractice lawsuits to determine if that level was maintained.
- Nurses should refuse to practice beyond the legal scope of practice and/or outside of their areas of competence regardless of reason (staffing shortage, lack of appropriate personnel).
- Nurses should use the formal chain of command to verbalize concerns related to assignment in light of current legal scope of practice, job description, and area of competence.

IMPAIRED COWORKERS

- Impaired health care providers pose a significant risk to client safety. Qs
- A nurse who suspects a coworker of using alcohol or other substances while working has a duty to report the coworker to appropriate management personnel as specified by institutional policy. At the time of the infraction, the report should be made to the immediate supervisor (the charge nurse, to ensure client safety).
- Health care facility policies should provide guidelines for handling employees who have a substance use disorder. Many facilities provide peer assistance programs that facilitate entry into a treatment program.
- Each state board of nursing has laws and regulations that govern the disposition of nurses who have been reported secondary to substance use. Depending on the individual case, the boards have the option to require the nurse to enter a treatment program, during which time the nurse's license can be retained, suspended, or revoked. If a nurse is allowed to maintain licensure, there usually are work restrictions put in place (working in noncritical care areas and being restricted from administering controlled medications).

- Health care providers who are found guilty of misappropriation of controlled substances also can be charged with a criminal offense consistent with the infraction.
- Behaviors can be difficult to detect if the impaired nurse is experienced at masking the substance use disorder.

BEHAVIORS CONSISTENT WITH A SUBSTANCE USE DISORDER

- Smell of alcohol on breath or frequent use of strong mouthwash or mints
- Impaired coordination, sleepiness, shakiness, and/or slurred speech
- Bloodshot eyes
- Mood swings and memory loss
- Neglect of personal appearance
- Excessive use of sick leave, tardiness, or absences after a weekend off, holiday, or payday
- Frequent requests to leave the unit for short periods of time or to leave the shift early
- Frequently "forgetting" to have another nurse witness wasting of a controlled substance
- Frequent involvement in incidences where a client assigned to the nurse reports not receiving pain medication or adequate pain relief (impaired nurse provides questionable explanations)
- Documenting administration of pain medication to a client who did not receive it or documenting a higher dosage than has been given by other nurses
- Preferring to work the night shift where supervision is less or on units where controlled substances are more frequently given

3.2 Elements necessary to prove negligence

		EXAMPLE: CLIENT WHO IS A FALL RISK
1.	*Duty to provide care as defined by a standard* Care that should be given or what a reasonably prudent nurse would do	The nurse should complete a fall risk assessment for all clients upon admission, per facility protocol.
2.	*Breach of duty by failure to meet standard* Failure to give the standard of care that should have been given	The nurse does not perform a fall risk assessment during admission.
3.	*Foreseeability of harm* Knowledge that failing to give the proper standard of care can cause harm to the client	The nurse should know that failure to take fall-risk precautions can endanger a client at risk for falls.
4.	*Breach of duty has potential to cause harm (combines elements 2 and 3)* Failure to meet the standard had potential to cause harm: relationship must be provable	If a fall risk assessment is not performed, the client's risk for falls is not determined and the proper precautions are not put in place.
5.	*Harm occurs* Occurrence of actual harm to the client	The client falls out of bed and breaks their hip.

MANDATORY REPORTING

In certain situations, health care providers have a legal obligation to report their findings in accordance with state law.

ABUSE

- All 51 jurisdictions (50 states and the District of Colombia) have statutes requiring report of suspicion of child abuse. The statutes set out which occupations are mandatory reporters. In many states, nurses are mandatory reporters.
- A number of states also mandate that health care providers, including nurses, report suspected violence of neglect against vulnerable persons (older or dependent adults).
- Nurses are mandated to report any suspicion of mistreatment following facility policy.

COMMUNICABLE DISEASES

- Nurses are also mandated to report to the proper agency (local health department, state health department) when a client is diagnosed with a communicable disease. Qs
- A complete list of reportable diseases and a description of the reporting system are available through the Centers for Disease Control and Prevention Web site. Each state mandates which diseases must be reported in that state. There are more than 60 communicable diseases that must be reported to public health departments to allow officials to do the following.
  - Ensure appropriate medical treatment of diseases (tuberculosis).
  - Monitor for common-source outbreaks (foodborne: hepatitis A).
  - Plan and evaluate control and prevention plans (immunizations for preventable diseases).
  - Identify outbreaks and epidemics.
  - Determine public health priorities based on trends.
  - Educate the community on prevention and treatment of these diseases.

ORGAN DONATION

- Organ and tissue donation is regulated by federal and state laws. Health care facilities have policies and procedures to guide health care workers involved with organ donation.
- Donations can be stipulated in a will or designated on an official card.
- Federal law requires health care facilities to provide access to trained specialists who make the request to clients and/or family members and provide information regarding consent, organ and tissues that can be donated, and how burial or cremation will be affected by donation.
- Nurses are responsible for answering questions regarding the donation process and for providing emotional support to family members.

TRANSCRIBING MEDICAL PRESCRIPTIONS

- Nurses might need to receive new prescriptions for client care or medications by verbal or telephone prescription.
- When transcribing a prescription into a paper or electronic chart, nurses must do the following.
  - Be sure to include all necessary elements of a prescription: date and time prescription was written; new client care prescription or medication including dosage, frequency, route of administration; and signature of nurse transcribing the prescription as well as the provider who verbally gave the prescription.
  - Follow institutional policy with regard to the time frame within which the provider must sign the prescription (usually within 24 hr).
  - Use strategies to prevent errors when taking a medical prescription that is given verbally or over the phone by the provider.
    - Repeat back the prescription given, making sure to include the medication name (spell if necessary), dosage, time, and route. Qs
    - Question any prescription that seems contraindicated due to a previous or concurrent prescription or client condition.

Disruptive behavior

- Nurses experience incivility, lateral violence, and bullying at an alarming rate. The perpetrator can be a provider or a nursing colleague. Consequences of disruptive behavior include poor communication, which can negatively affect client safety and productivity, resulting in absenteeism, decreased job satisfaction, and staff turnover. Some nurses can choose to leave the profession due to these counterproductive behaviors.
- If disruptive behavior is allowed to continue, it is likely to escalate. Over time, it can be viewed as acceptable in that unit or department's culture.

TYPES OF DISRUPTIVE BEHAVIOR

- **Incivility** is defined as an action that is rude, intimidating, and insulting. It includes teasing, joking, dirty looks, and uninvited touching.
- **Lateral violence** is also known as horizontal abuse or horizontal hostility. It occurs between individuals who are at the same level within the organization. For example, a more experienced staff nurse can be abusive to a newly licensed nurse. Common behaviors include verbal abuse, undermining activities, sabotage, gossip, withholding information, and ostracism.
- **Bullying** behavior is persistent and relentless and is aimed at an individual who has limited ability to defend themselves. Bullying occurs when the perpetrator is at a higher level than the victim (for example, a nurse manager to a staff nurse). It is abuse of power that makes the recipient feel threatened, disgraced, and vulnerable. For example, a nurse manager can demonstrate favoritism for another nurse by making unfair assignments or refusing a promotion.
- **Cyberbullying** is a type of disruptive behavior using the Internet or other electronic means.

INTERVENTIONS TO DETER DISRUPTIVE BEHAVIORS

- Create an environment of mutual respect among staff.
- Model appropriate behavior.
- Increase staff awareness about disruptive behavior.
- Make staff aware that offensive online remarks about employers and coworkers are a form of bullying and are prohibited even if the nurse is off-duty and it is posted off-site from the facility.
- Avoid making excuses for disruptive behavior.
- Support zero tolerance for disruptive behavior.
- Establish mechanisms for open communication between staff nurses and nurse managers.
- Adopt policies that limit the risk of retaliation when disruptive behavior is reported.

Ethical practice

- **Ethics** has several definitions, but the foundation of ethics is based on an expected behavior of a certain group in relation to what is considered right and wrong.
- **Morals** are the values and beliefs held by a person that guide behavior and decision-making.
- **Ethical theory** analyzes varying philosophies, systems, ideas, and principles used to make judgments about what is right and wrong, good and bad. Two common types of ethical theory are utilitarianism and deontology.
  - Utilitarianism (teleological theory): Decision-making based on what provides the greatest good for the greatest number of individuals
  - Deontological theory: Decision-making based on obligations, duty, and what one considers to be right or wrong
- Unusual or complex ethical issues might need to be dealt with by a facility's ethics committee.

ETHICAL PRINCIPLES are standards of what is right or wrong with regard to important social values and norms. Ethical principles pertaining to the treatment of clients include the following. Qpcc
- **Autonomy:** The ability of the client to make personal decisions, even when those decisions might not be in the client's own best interest
- **Beneficence:** Care that is in the best interest of the client
- **Fidelity:** Keeping one's promise to the client about care that was offered
- **Justice:** Fair treatment in matters related to physical and psychosocial care and use of resources
- **Nonmaleficence:** The nurse's obligation to avoid causing harm to the client
- **Veracity:** The nurse's duty to tell the truth

ETHICAL DECISION-MAKING IN NURSING

Ethical dilemmas are problems for which more than one choice can be made, and the choice is influenced by the values and beliefs of the decision-makers. These are common in health care, and nurses must be prepared to apply ethical theory and decision-making.

- A problem is an ethical dilemma if:
  - It cannot be solved solely by a review of scientific data.
  - It involves a conflict between two moral imperatives.
  - The answer will have a profound effect on the situation/client.
- Nurses have a responsibility to be advocates, and to identify and report ethical situations.
  - Doing so through the chain of command offers some protection against retribution.
  - Some state nurse associations offer protection for nurses who report substandard or unethical practice.
- Ethical decision-making is the process by which a decision is made about an ethical issue. Frequently, this requires a balance between science and morality. There are several steps in ethical decision-making:
  - Identify whether the issue is an ethical dilemma.
  - State the ethical dilemma, including all surrounding issues and individuals involved.
  - List and analyze all possible options for resolving the dilemma, and review implications of each option.
  - Select the option that is in concert with the ethical principle applicable to this situation, the decision maker's values and beliefs, and the profession's values set forth for client care. Justify why that one option was selected.
  - Apply this decision to the dilemma and evaluate the outcomes.
- The American Nurses Association Code of Ethics for Nurses and the International Council of Nurses' Code of Ethics for Nurses are commonly used by professional nurses. The Code of Ethics for Licensed Practical/Vocational Nurses issued by the National Association for Practical Nurse Education and Services also serves as a set of standards for Nursing Practice. Codes of ethics are available at the organizations' websites.
- The Uniform Determination of Death Act (UDDA) can be used to assist with end-of-life and organ donor issues.
  - The UDDA provides two formal definitions of death that were developed by the National Conference of Commissioners on Uniform State Laws. Death is determined by one of two criteria.
    - Irreversible cessation of circulatory and respiratory functions
    - Irreversible cessation of all functions of the entire brain, including the brain stem
  - A determination of death must be made in accordance with accepted medical standards.

3.3 The nurse's role in ethical decision-making

	EXAMPLES
An agent for the client facing an ethical decision	Caring for an adolescent client who is deciding whether to undergo an elective abortion even though their parents believe it is wrong
	Discussing options with parents who have to decide whether to consent to a blood transfusion for a child when their religion prohibits such treatment
A decision-maker in regard to nursing practice	Assigning staff nurses a higher client load than recommended because administration has cut the number of nurses per shift
	Witnessing a surgeon discuss only surgical options with a client without informing the client about more conservative measures available

Active Learning Scenario

A nurse is preparing to serve on a committee that will review the policy on disruptive behavior. Use the ATI Active Learning Template: Basic Concept to complete this item.

RELATED CONTENT: Describe another term used for lateral violence.

NURSING INTERVENTIONS: Describe at least four interventions to deter disruptive behavior.

Active Learning Scenario Key

Using the ATI Active Learning Template: Basic Concept

RELATED CONTENT: Lateral violence is also known as horizontal abuse or horizontal hostility.

NURSING INTERVENTIONS
- Create an environment of mutual respect among staff.
- Model appropriate behavior.
- Increase staff awareness about disruptive behavior.
- Make staff aware that offensive online remarks about employers and coworkers are a form of bullying and is prohibited even if the nurse is off-duty and it is posted off-site of the facility.
- Avoid making excuses for disruptive behavior.
- Support zero tolerance for disruptive behavior.
- Establish mechanisms for open communication between staff nurses and nurse managers.
- Adopt policies that limit the risk of retaliation when disruptive behavior is reported.

Ⓝ *NCLEX® Connection: Management of Care, Concepts of Management*

Application Exercises

1. A nurse manager is observing the actions of a nurse they are supervising. Which of the following actions by the nurse requires the nurse manager to intervene? (Select all that apply.)

   A. Reviewing the health care record of a client assigned to another nurse

   B. Making a copy of a client's most current laboratory results for the provider during rounds

   C. Providing information about a client's condition to hospital clergy

   D. Discussing a client's condition over the phone with an individual who has provided the client's information code

   E. Participating in walking rounds that involve the exchange of client-related information outside clients' rooms

2. A nurse is caring for a client who is scheduled for surgery. The client hands the nurse information about advance directives and states, "Here, I don't need this. I am too young to worry about life-sustaining measures and what I want done for me." Which of the following actions should the nurse take?

   A. Return the papers to the admitting department with a note stating that the client does not wish to address the issue at this time.

   B. Explain to the client that you never know what can happen during surgery and to fill the papers out just in case.

   C. Contact a client representative to talk with the client and offer additional information about the purpose of advance directives.

   D. Inform the client that surgery cannot be conducted unless the advance directives forms are completed.

3. A nurse witnesses an assistive personnel (AP) they are supervising reprimanding a client for not using the urinal properly. The AP threatens to put a diaper on the client if the urinal is not used more carefully next time. Which of the following torts is the AP committing?

   A. Assault

   B. Battery

   C. False imprisonment

   D. Invasion of privacy

4. A nurse is serving as a preceptor to a newly licensed nurse and is explaining the role of the nurse as advocate. Which of the following situations illustrates the advocacy role? (Select all that apply.)

   A. Verifying that a client understands what is done during a cardiac catheterization

   B. Discussing treatment options for a terminal diagnosis

   C. Informing members of the health care team that a client has do-not-resuscitate status

   D. Reporting that a health team member on the previous shift did not provide care as prescribed

   E. Assisting a client to make a decision about their care based on the nurse's recommendations

5. A nurse manager is providing information to the nurses on the unit about ensuring client rights. Which of the following regulations outlines the rights of individuals in health care settings?

   A. American Nurses Association Code of Ethics

   B. HIPAA

   C. Patient Self-Determination Act

   D. Patient Care Partnership

6. A newly licensed nurse is preparing to insert an IV catheter in a client. Which of the following sources should the nurse use to review the procedure and the standard at which it should be performed?

   A. Website

   B. Institutional policy and procedure manual

   C. More experienced nurse

   D. State nurse practice act

7. A nurse is caring for a client who is medically unstable. The client's adult child informs the nurse that the client has a DNR prescription with their primary care provider. Which of the following actions should the nurse take?

   A. Assume that the client does not want to be resuscitated, and take no action if they experience cardiac arrest.

   B. Write a note on the front of the provider prescription sheet asking that the DNR be represcribed.

   C. Write a DNR prescription in the client's medical record.

   D. Call the provider to verify the existence of an active DNR prescription.

8. A nurse is caring for a child who is being treated in the emergency department following a head contusion from a fall. History reveals the child lives at home with one parent. The provider's discharge instructions include waking the child every hour to assess for indications of a possible head injury. In which of the following situations should the nurse intervene and attempt to prevent discharge?

   A. The parent states they do not have insurance or money for a follow-up visit.

   B. The child states, "My head hurts and I want to go home."

   C. The nurse smells alcohol on the parent's breath.

   D. The parent verbalizes fear about taking the child home and requests they be kept overnight.

Application Exercises Key

1. A. **CORRECT:** To maintain confidentiality, client information is disseminated on a need-to-know basis only. A nurse who is not assigned to care for a client should not access the client's information.
   B. **CORRECT:** Paper copies of confidential information create a risk for breach of confidentiality.
   C. **CORRECT:** Information about a client's condition is disseminated on a need-to-know basis. It is inappropriate to share this information with the hospital clergy.
   D. The nurse can share information with an individual who has been provided the information code.
   E. **CORRECT:** Sharing information in the hallway where it can be overheard by others can result in a breach of confidentiality.

   Ⓝ *NCLEX® Connection: Management of Care, Assignment, Delegation and Supervision*

2. A. The nurse should advocate for the client by ensuring that the client understands the purpose of advance directives.
   B. This response is nontherapeutic and can cause the client to be anxious about the surgery.
   C. **CORRECT:** The nurse should advocate for the client by ensuring that the client understands the purpose of advance directives. Seeking the assistance of a client representative to provide information to the client is an appropriate action.
   D. This statement is untrue and is a barrier to therapeutic communication.

   Ⓝ *NCLEX® Connection: Management of Care, Advance Directives/Self-Determine/Life Planning*

3. A. **CORRECT:** Assault is conduct that makes a person fear they will be harmed.
   B. Battery is physical contact without a person's consent.
   C. False imprisonment is restraining a person against their will. It includes the use of physical or chemical restraints, and refusing to allow a client to leave a facility.
   D. Invasion of privacy is the unauthorized release of a client's private information.

   Ⓝ *NCLEX® Connection: Management of Care, Concepts of Management*

4. A. **CORRECT:** Ensuring that the client has given informed consent illustrates nurse advocacy.
   B. Discussing treatment options is not within the scope of practice of the nurse.
   C. **CORRECT:** Ensuring that the client's care is consistent with their DNR status illustrates nurse advocacy.
   D. **CORRECT:** Ensuring that all clients receive proper care illustrates nurse advocacy.
   E. Assisting a client to make decisions about their care based on nurse recommendations is inappropriate. The nurse should support the client in making their own decisions.

   Ⓝ *NCLEX® Connection: Management of Care, Client Rights*

5. A. The American Nurses Association Code of Ethics provides nurses with a set of standards for nursing practice.
   B. The Privacy Rule of HIPAA ensures client privacy and confidentiality.
   C. The Patient Self-Determination Act is federal legislation that requires that all clients admitted to a health care facility be asked whether they have advance directives.
   D. **CORRECT:** The Patient Care Partnership is a document that addresses clients' rights when receiving care.

   Ⓝ *NCLEX® Connection: Management of Care, Information Technology*

6. A. A website might not provide information that is consistent with institutional policy.
   B. **CORRECT:** The institutional policy and procedure manual will provide instructions on how to perform the procedure that is consistent with established standards. This is the resource that should be used.
   C. A more experienced nurse on the unit might not perform the procedure according to the policy and procedure manual.
   D. The nurse practice act identifies scope of practice and other aspects of the law, but it does not set standards for performance of a procedure.

   Ⓝ *NCLEX® Connection: Management of Care, Advance Directives/Self-Determine/Life Planning*

7. A. Without a current DNR prescription, the nurse must initiate emergency resuscitation, which most likely is not consistent with the client's wishes.
   B. Without a current DNR prescription, the nurse must initiate emergency resuscitation, which most likely is not consistent with the client's wishes. Writing a note on the prescription sheet likely will result in a delay in resolving the problem.
   C. The nurse cannot write a DNR prescription for the client without instruction to do so by the primary provider.
   D. **CORRECT:** The nurse should immediately call the primary provider to validate whether the client has a current DNR order in place.

   Ⓝ *NCLEX® Connection: Management of Care, Advocacy*

8. A. Lack of insurance does not warrant a delay in discharge, but it can indicate the need for referral for social services to assist with client needs.
   B. The child's report of pain is an expected finding.
   C. **CORRECT:** It would be unsafe to discharge a child who requires hourly monitoring with a parent who might be chemically impaired.
   D. Fear verbalized by the parent does not warrant denial in discharge. The nurse should alleviate the parent's fears by providing education about how to monitor the child and provide phone numbers for use.

   Ⓝ *NCLEX® Connection: Management of Care, Ethical Practice*

When reviewing the following chapter, keep in mind the relevant topics and tasks of the NCLEX outline, in particular:

Safety and Infection Control

ACCIDENT/ERROR/INJURY PREVENTION: Determine client/staff member knowledge of safety procedures.

CASE MANAGEMENT: Initiate, evaluate, and update client plan of care.

CONTINUITY OF CARE
Perform procedures necessary to safely admit, transfer and/pr discharge a client.

Follow up on unresolved issues regarding client care (e.g., laboratory results, client requests).

STANDARD PRECAUTIONS/TRANSMISSION-BASED PRECAUTIONS/SURGICAL ASEPSIS: Educate client and staff regarding infection control measures.

Maintaining a Safe Environment

CHAPTER 4

Maintaining a safe environment refers to the precautions and considerations required to ensure that physical environments are safe for clients and staff. Qs

Knowing how to maintain client safety has been identified by the Institute of Medicine as a competency that graduates of nursing programs must possess.

Common errors in health care are related to medication errors, errors related to diagnostic testing, surgical errors, health care-acquired infection, and errors in hand-off reporting and care.

Quality and Safety Education for Nurses (QSEN) faculty propose that nursing education focus not only on the knowledge needed to provide safe care but also on the skills and attitudes that accompany this competency.

To maintain a safe environment, nurses must have knowledge, skills, and attitudes about QSEN competencies, handling infectious and hazardous materials, safe use of equipment, accident and injury prevention, home safety, and ergonomic principles.

Culture of safety

- A culture of safety is one that promotes openness and error reporting. Developing a culture of safety often results in a lower number of adverse events.
- Facilities should have a risk management department to help identify and prevent adverse events, hazards, track the occurrence of negative client incidents, and help manage the hazards.
- There are several types of events that are reported and tracked under risk management programs.

Service occurrences relate to client services, and can include a slight delay in service or an unsatisfactory service.

Near misses are situations where a negative outcome almost occurs (an accident, illness, or injury.

Serious incidents reported include minor injuries, loss of equipment or property, or a significant service interrupted.

Sentinel events refer to unexpected death or major injury, whether physical or psychological, or situations where there was a direct risk of either of these. Major investigation is required in the case of sentinel events. Sentinel events are classified as one of the following.
- Major loss of function or death that was not expected with the client's medical condition
- Client attempted suicide during round-the-clock care, a hemolytic transfusion reaction, wrong site or wrong client surgical procedures, rape, infant abduction, or discharge to the wrong family.

Failure to rescue is the most severe, and describes a situation where the client develops a complication that leads to death. In failure to rescue situations, there were client indicators that were missed by one or more health care personnel that indicated that a complication was occurring.

QSEN competencies in nursing programs

Concern about the quality and safety of health care in the U.S. has prompted numerous reports and initiatives designed to address this issue. Data from the Joint Commission identify poor communication as a key factor in the majority of sentinel events. The Institute of Medicine (IOM) report *To Err is Human: Building a Safer Health System* (1999) spoke to the frequency of unnecessary deaths and preventable medical errors, and identified system failure as a major factor. Subsequent publications pointed to the need to redesign the provision of client care and improve education of students in health care programs.

The QSEN project identified specific competencies to include in each prelicensure nursing curriculum. These six competencies are now integral components of the curriculum of many nursing programs in the U.S.

Qᴾᶜᶜ PATIENT-CENTERED CARE: The provision of caring and compassionate, culturally sensitive care that addresses clients' physiological, psychological, sociological, spiritual, and cultural needs, preferences, and values

Qᵀᶜ TEAMWORK AND COLLABORATION: The delivery of client care in partnership with multidisciplinary members of the health care team to achieve continuity of care and positive client outcomes

Qᴱᴮᴾ EVIDENCE-BASED PRACTICE: The use of current knowledge from research and other credible sources on which to base clinical judgment and client care

Qᵠᴵ QUALITY IMPROVEMENT: Care-related and organizational processes that involve the development and implementation of a plan to improve health care services and better meet clients' needs

Qˢ SAFETY: The minimization of risk factors that could cause injury or harm while promoting quality care and maintaining a secure environment for clients, self, and others

Qᴵ INFORMATICS: The use of information technology as a communication and information-gathering tool that supports clinical decision-making and scientifically-based nursing practice

Handling infectious and hazardous materials

- Handling infectious and hazardous materials refers to infection control procedures and to precautions for handling toxic, radioactive, or other hazardous materials. Qˢ
- Safety measures are taken to protect the client, nurse, and other personnel and individuals from harmful materials and organisms.

INFECTION CONTROL

Infection control is extremely important to prevent cross-contamination of communicable organisms and health care-associated infections.
- Staff education on infection prevention and control is a responsibility of the nurse.
- Facility policies and procedures should serve as a resource for proper implementation of infection prevention and control.
- Clients suspected of having or known to have a communicable disease should be placed in the appropriate form of isolation.
- The nurse should ensure that appropriate equipment is available and that isolation procedures are properly carried out by all health care team members.
- Use of standard precautions by all members of the health care team should be enforced. Employees who are allergic to latex should have non-latex gloves (nitrile or vinyl) made available to them. A latex-free environment is provided for clients who have a latex allergy. Many facilities avoid the use of latex products unless there is no other alternative.
- Facilities should provide resources for employees to perform hand hygiene in client care areas.
- Use moisture-resistant bags for disposing of soiled items, tied securely. To remain cost-effective, only double-bag if the outside of a bag becomes contaminated.
- Use safety needles or needless IV systems to prevent care and staff injuries from improper manipulation.
- Dispose of sharps in sharps containers immediately after use.
- If a needlestick occurs, report it to facility risk management in accordance with facility policy and state law. An incident or occurrence report should also be filed. Most policies include testing of the client and nurse for bloodborne illnesses (hepatitis and human immunodeficiency virus [HIV]).
- Four levels of precautions (standard, airborne, droplet, contact) are recommended for individuals coming in contact with clients carrying infectious organisms. Precautions consistent with the infectious organism should be followed as indicated.
- Members of the health care team must clean and maintain equipment that is shared by clients on a unit (blood pressure cuffs, thermometers, pulse oximeters).
- Keep designated equipment in the rooms of clients who are on contact precautions.

HAZARDOUS MATERIALS

- Nurses and other members of the health care team are at risk for exposure to hazardous materials.
- Employees have the right to refuse to work in hazardous working conditions if there is a clear threat to their health.
- Health care team members should follow occupational safety and health guidelines as set by the Occupational Safety and Health Administration (OSHA).
  - Provide each employee a work environment that is free from recognized hazards that can cause or are likely to cause death or serious physical harm.
  - Make protective gear accessible to employees working under hazardous conditions or with hazardous materials (antineoplastic medications, sterilization chemicals).
  - Provide measurement devices and keeping records that document an employee's level of exposure over time to hazardous materials (radiation from x-rays).
  - Provide education and recertification opportunities to each employee regarding these rules and regulations (handling of hazardous materials).
  - A manual containing safety data sheets (SDSs) should be available in every workplace and provide safety information (level of toxicity, handling and storage guidelines, and first aid and containment measures to take in case of accidental release of toxic, radioactive, or other dangerous materials). This manual should be available to all employees and can be housed in a location (the emergency department of a hospital).
  - Designate an institutional hazardous materials (HAZMAT) response team that responds to hazardous events.

Safe use of equipment

Safe use of equipment refers to the appropriate operation of health care-related equipment by trained staff. Equipment-related injuries can occur as a result of malfunction, disrepair, or mishandling of mechanical equipment. Qs

Nurses' responsibilities related to equipment safety

- Learning how to use and maintaining competency in the use of equipment
- Checking that equipment is accurately set and functioning properly (oxygen, nasogastric suction) at the beginning and during each shift
- Ensuring that electrical equipment is grounded (three-pronged plug and grounded outlet) to decrease the risk for electrical shock
- Ensuring that outlet covers are used in environments with individuals at risk for sticking items into them
- Unplugging equipment using the plug, not the cord, to prevent bending the plug prongs, which increases the risk for electrical shock
- Ensuring that life-support equipment is plugged into outlets designated to be powered by a backup generator during power outages
- Disconnecting all electrical equipment prior to cleaning

- Ensuring that all pumps (general and PCA) have free-flow protection to prevent an overdose of fluids or medications
- Ensuring that outlets are not overcrowded and that extension cords are used only when absolutely necessary (if they must be used in an open area, tape the cords to the floor)
- Using all equipment only as it is intended
- Equipment should be regularly inspected by the engineering or maintenance department and by the user prior to use. Faulty equipment (frayed cords, disrepair) can start a fire or cause an electrical shock and should be removed from use and reported immediately per agency policy.

Specific risk areas

- Preventing injury is a major nursing responsibility.
- Many factors affect a client's ability to protect themselves. Qs
  - Age (pediatric and older adult clients are at greater risk)
  - Mobility
  - Cognitive and sensory awareness
  - Emotional state
  - Lifestyle and safety awareness
- Review facility protocol for managing specific high-risk situations.

FALLS

Prevention of client falls is a major nursing priority. Screen all clients for risk factors related to falls.

- Physiological changes associated with aging (decreased strength, impaired mobility and balance, endurance limitations, decreased sensory perception) can increase the risk of injury for some older adults. Ⓖ
- To evaluate incidence of client falls, a formula based on 1,000 client days can be used. Using this formula, a facility can compare its fall rates to other facilities.

(Number of client falls ÷ number of client days) × 1,000 = fall rate per 1,000 client days

- Other risk factors include decreased visual acuity, generalized weakness, orthopedic problems (diabetic neuropathy), urinary frequency, gait and balance problems (Parkinson's disease, osteoporosis, arthritis), and cognitive dysfunction. Adverse effects of medications (orthostatic hypotension, drowsiness) also can increase the risk for falls.
- Clients are at greater risk for falls when multiple risk factors are present, and clients who have fallen previously are at risk for falling again.

PREVENTION OF FALLS Qs

The plan for each client is individualized based on the fall risk assessment findings.

GENERAL MEASURES TO PREVENT FALLS
- Ensure that the client understands how to use all assistive devices and can locate necessary items.
- Place clients at risk for falls near the nursing station.
- Ensure that bedside tables, overbed tables, and frequently used items (telephone, water, tissues, call light) are within the client's reach.
- Maintain the bed in low position.
- Keep bed rails up for clients who are sedated, unconscious, or otherwise compromised, and partly up for other clients.
- Avoid using full side bed rails for clients who get out of bed or attempt to get out of bed without assistance.
- Provide the client with nonskid footwear.
- Keep the floor free from clutter with a clear path to the bathroom (no scatter rugs, cords, furniture).
- Ensure adequate lighting.
- Lock wheels on beds, wheelchairs, and carts to prevent the device from rolling during transfers or stops.
- Use chair or bed sensors to alert staff of independent ambulation for clients at risk for getting up unattended.

SEIZURES

Seizures can occur at any time during a person's life and can be due to epilepsy, fever, or a variety of medical conditions.

SEIZURE PRECAUTIONS

Seizure precautions (measures to protect the client from injury should a seizure occur) are taken for clients who have a history of seizures that involve the entire body or result in unconsciousness. Qs
- Protective measures for clients who are at high risk for a seizure include assigning the client a room close to the nurses station and inserting a peripheral IV.
- Ensure that rescue equipment, including oxygen, an oral airway, and suction equipment, is at the bedside. A saline lock can be placed for intravenous access if the client is at high risk for experiencing a generalized seizure.
- Instruct the client to use precautions when out of bed.
- If a seizure occurs, provide monitoring and treatment as indicated. **SEE FUNDAMENTALS CHAPTER 12: CLIENT SAFETY.**

SECLUSION AND RESTRAINTS

Seclusion and restraints are used to prevent clients from injuring themselves or others. **FOR MORE ABOUT RESTRAINTS, SEE FUNDAMENTALS CHAPTER 12: CLIENT SAFETY.**
- Seclusion is the placement of a client in a room that is, and safe. Seclusion is used for clients who are at risk for injuring themselves or others.
- Physical restraint involves the application of a device that limits the client's movement. A restraint can limit the movement of the entire body or a body part.
- Chemical restraints are medications used to control the client's disruptive behavior.

RISKS ASSOCIATED WITH RESTRAINTS Qs

- Deaths by asphyxiation and strangulation have occurred with restraints. Many facilities no longer use a vest restraint for that reason.
- The client can also experience complications related to immobility (pressure injuries, urinary and fecal incontinence, pneumonia).

LEGAL CONSIDERATIONS

- Nurses should understand agency polices as well as federal and state laws that govern the use of restraints and seclusion.
- False imprisonment means the confinement of a person without their consent. Improper use of restraints can subject the nurse to charges of false imprisonment.

GUIDELINES

- Use restraints according to the prescription parameters, for the shortest time necessary. Attempt early release if the client behavior is calm.
- Restraints are for the protection of clients or others, after all other possible methods of behavior change have been tried.
- The client or family might feel embarrassed about the restraints. Explain the purpose of the restraint and that the restraint is only temporary.
- PRN prescriptions for restraints are not permitted.
- The treatment must be prescribed by the provider based on a face-to-face assessment of the client. In an emergency situation in which there is immediate risk to the client or others, the nurse can place a client in restraints. The nurse must obtain a prescription from the provider as soon as possible in accordance with agency policy (usually within 1 hr).
- The prescription must specify the reason for the restraint, the type of restraint, the location of the restraint, how long the restraint can be used, and the type of behaviors demonstrated by the client that warrant use of the restraint.
- In medical facilities, the prescription should be limited to 8 hr of restraints for an adult, 2 hr for clients age 9 to 17, and 1 hr for clients younger than 9 years of age. For adult clients who have violent or self-destructive behavior, the prescription should be for 4 hr. Providers can renew these prescriptions with a maximum of 24 consecutive hours.

NURSING RESPONSIBILITIES

Obtain a prescription from the provider for the restraint. If the client is at risk for harming self or others and a restraint is applied prior to consulting the provider, ensure that notification of the provider occurs in accordance with facility protocol

- Conduct neurosensory checks every 2 hr or according to facility policy to include:
  - Circulation.
  - Sensation
  - Mobility
- Offer food and fluids.
- Provide with means for hygiene and elimination.
- Monitor vital signs.
- Provide range of motion of extremities.
- Follow agency polices regarding restraints, including the need for signed consent from the client or guardian.
- Review the manufacturer's instructions for correct application.
- Remove or replace restraints frequently.
- Pad bony prominences.
- Secure restraints to a movable part of the bed frame. If restraints with a buckle strap are not available, use a quick-release knot to tie the strap.
- Ensure that the restraint is loose enough for range of motion and has enough room to fit two fingers between the device and the client.
- Regularly assess the need for continued use of restraints.
- Never leave the client unattended without the restraint.
- Document client data before, during, and after restraint use, as well as behavioral interventions and care measures.

FIRE SAFETY

Fires in health care facilities are usually due to problems related to electrical or anesthetic equipment. Unauthorized smoking can also be the cause of a fire.

All staff must:
- Know the location of exits, alarms, fire extinguishers, and oxygen turnoff valves.
- Make sure equipment does not block fire doors.
- Know the evacuation plan for the unit and the facility.

Fire response follows the RACE sequence

R: Rescue and protect clients in close proximity to the fire by moving them to a safer location. Clients who are ambulatory can walk independently to a safe location.

A: Alarm: Activate the facility's alarm system and then report the fire's details and location.

C: Confine the fire by closing doors and windows and turning off any sources of oxygen and any electrical devices. Ventilate clients who are on life support with a bag-valve mask.

E: Extinguish the fire if possible using the appropriate fire extinguisher.

FIRE EXTINGUISHERS

To use a fire extinguisher, use the PASS sequence.

P: Pull the pin.

A: Aim at the base of the fire.

S: Squeeze the handle.

S: Sweep the extinguisher from side to side, covering the area of the fire.

Classes of fire extinguishers

Class A is for combustibles (paper, wood, upholstery, rags, and other types of trash fires).

Class B is for flammable liquids and gas fires.

Class C is for electrical fires.

Home safety

Nurses play a pivotal role in promoting safety in the client's home and community. Nurses often collaborate with the client, family, and members of the interprofessional team (social workers, occupational therapists, physical therapists) to promote client safety. Qтᴄ

When the client demonstrates factors that increases the risk for injury (regardless of age), a home hazard evaluation should be conducted by a nurse, physical therapist, and/or occupational therapist. The client is made aware of the environmental factors that can pose a risk to safety and suggested modifications to be made.

Many factors contribute to the client's risk for injury.
- Age and developmental status
- Mobility and balance
- Knowledge about safety hazards
- Sensory and cognitive awareness
- Communication skills
- Home and work environment
- Community
- Medical and pharmacological status

To initiate a plan of care, the nurse must identify risk factors using a risk assessment tool and complete a nursing history, physical examination, and home hazard appraisal.

SAFETY RISKS BASED ON AGE AND DEVELOPMENTAL STATUS

- The age and developmental status of the client create specific safety risks. QPCC
- Infants and toddlers are at risk for injury due to a tendency to put objects in their mouth and from hazards encountered while exploring their environment.
- Preschool- and school-age children often face injury from limited or underdeveloped motor coordination.
- Adolescents' risks for injury can stem from increased desire to make independent decisions, and relying on peers for guidance rather than family.
- Some of the accident prevention measures for specific age groups are found below. **SEE FUNDAMENTALS CHAPTER 13: HOME SAFETY FOR AGE-SPECIFIC SAFETY RECOMMENDATIONS.**

INFANTS AND TODDLERS

Aspiration
- Keep all small objects out of reach.
- Cut or break food that is age-appropriate into small bite-size pieces.
- Do not place the infant in the supine position while feeding or to prop the infant's bottle.

Water safety
- Never leave an infant or toddler unattended in the bathtub.
- Block access to bathrooms, pools, and other standing water.
- Begin teaching water safety when developmentally appropriate.

Suffocation
- Follow recommendations for safe sleep environment and positioning for infants.
- Keep latex balloons and plastic bags away from infants and toddlers.
- Teach caregivers CPR and Heimlich maneuver.

Poisoning
- Keep houseplants and cleaning agents locked away and out of reach.
- Inspect for and remove chemicals, medications, and sources of lead.

Falls
- Prevent falls from cribs, high beds, diaper changing surfaces, stairs, and windows.
- Restrain according to manufacturer's recommendations and supervise when in a high chair, swing, stroller, etc. Discontinue use when the infant or toddler outgrows size limits.

Motor vehicle injury
- Follow car seat requirements based on height, weight, and age.
- Follow recommendations for choosing a safe car seat, and always place it in the back seat.

Burns
- Supervise the use of faucets and test water temperature.
- Keep matches, lighters, and electrical equipment and sources out of reach.

PRESCHOOLERS AND SCHOOL-AGE CHILDREN

Drowning
- Be sure the child has learned to swim and knows rules of water safety.
- Prevent unsupervised access to pools or other bodies of water.
- Teach wearing a life jacket in boats.

Motor vehicle injury
- Follow recommendations for car seat use and placement.
- Use seat belts properly after booster seats are no longer necessary.
- Use protective equipment when participating in sports, riding a bike, or riding as a passenger on a bike.
- Teach the child safety rules of the road.

Firearms
- Keep firearms unloaded, locked up, and out of reach.
- Teach to never touch a gun or stay at a friend's house where a gun is accessible.
- Store bullets in a different location from guns.

Play injury
- Ensure that play equipment are the appropriate size for the child.
- Teach to play in safe areas, and avoid heavy machinery, railroad tracks, excavation areas, quarries, trunks, vacant buildings, and empty refrigerators.
- Teach to avoid strangers and keep parents informed of strangers.

Burns
- Teach dangers of playing with matches, fireworks, and firearms.
- Teach school-age child how to properly use a microwave and other cooking instruments.

Poison
- Teach the child about the hazards of alcohol, cigarettes, and prescription, non-prescription, and illegal substances.
- Keep potentially dangerous substances out of reach.
- Teach parents to have the nationwide poison control number near every phone in the home and programmed in each cell phone (1-800-222-1222).

ADOLESCENTS

Motor vehicle and injury
- Ensure the teen has completed a driver's education course.
- Set rules on the number of people allowed to ride in cars, seat belt use, and to call for a ride home if a driver is impaired.
- Reinforce safety precautions for sports and hobbies.
- Teach water safety.

Burns
- Teach to use sunblock and protective clothing.
- Teach the dangers of sunbathing and tanning beds.

Other risks
- Be alert to indications of depression, anxiety, or other behavioral changes.
- Educate on the hazards of smoking, alcohol, legal and illegal substances, and unprotected sex.
- Discuss dangers of social networking and the Internet.

YOUNG AND MIDDLE-AGE ADULTS

Motor vehicle crashes are a leading cause of death and injury to adults. Occupational injuries contribute to the injury and death rate of adults. High consumption of alcohol and suicide are also major concerns for adults.

CLIENT EDUCATION
- Follow recommendations for safe alcohol consumption.
- Be attuned to behaviors that suggest the presence of depression or thoughts of suicide. Seek counseling or contact a provider.
- Be proactive about safety in the workplace and in the home.
- Be aware of hazards associated with networking and the Internet.
- Protect skin with the use of sun-blocking agents and protective clothing.

OLDER ADULTS

- Many older adults are able to maintain a lifestyle that promotes independence and the ability to protect themselves from safety hazards.
- Prevention is important because elderly clients can have longer recovery times from injuries and are at an increased risk for complications from injuries.

RISK FACTORS FOR FALLS
- The rate at which age-related changes occur varies greatly among older adults ©
- Physical, cognitive, and sensory changes
- Changes in the musculoskeletal and neurologic systems
- Impaired vision and/or hearing
- Ambulating frequently at night because of nocturia and incontinence

MODIFICATIONS TO IMPROVE HOME SAFETY
- Remove items that could cause the client to trip (throw rugs).
- Provide assistive devices and safety equipment.
- Ensure that lighting is adequate inside and outside the home.

HOME SAFETY PLAN

- Keep emergency numbers near the phone for prompt use in the event of an emergency of any type.
- Develop a family plan for evacuating the home and practice it regularly.

FIRE

Home fires continue to be a major cause of death and injury for people of all ages. Nurses should educate clients about the importance of a home safety plan.
- Ensure that the number and placement of fire extinguishers and smoke alarms are adequate and that they are operable.
- Be sure to close windows and doors if able.
- Exit a smoke-filled area by covering the mouth and nose with a damp cloth and getting down as close to the floor as possible.
- In the event that the clothing or skin is on fire, "stop, drop, and roll" to extinguish the fire.

SAFE USE OF OXYGEN IN THE HOME

If oxygen is used in the home, oxygen safety measures should be reviewed. Oxygen can cause materials to combust more easily and burn more rapidly, so the client and family must be provided with information on use of the oxygen delivery equipment and the dangers of combustion.
- Use and store oxygen equipment according to the manufacturer's recommendations.
- Place a "No Smoking" sign in a conspicuous place near the front door of the home. A sign can also be placed on the door to the client's bedroom.
- Inform the client and family of the danger of smoking in the presence of oxygen. Family members and visitors who smoke should do so outside the home.
- Ensure that electrical equipment is in good repair and well grounded.
- Replace bedding that generates static electricity (wool, nylon, synthetics) with items made from cotton.
- Keep flammable materials (heating oil and nail polish remover) away from the client when oxygen is in use.
- Follow general measures for fire safety in the home (having a fire extinguisher readily available and an established exit route) should a fire occur.

ADDITIONAL RISKS IN THE HOME AND COMMUNITY

Additional risks in the home and community include passive smoking, carbon monoxide poisoning, and food poisoning. Natural and human-made disasters are a threat to homes and communities. Nurses should teach clients about the dangers of these additional risks.

Passive smoking

Passive smoking (secondhand smoke) is the unintentional inhalation of tobacco smoke.

- Exposure to nicotine and other toxins places people at risk for numerous diseases, including cancer, heart disease, and lung infections.
- Low birth weight, prematurity, stillbirths, and sudden infant death syndrome (SIDS) have been associated with maternal smoking.
- Passive smoking is associated with childhood development of bronchitis, pneumonia, and middle ear infections.
- For children who have asthma, exposure to passive smoke can result in an increase in the frequency and the severity of asthma attacks.

NURSING ACTIONS

- Inform clients about the hazards of smoking and exposure to smoke from cigarettes, cigars, and pipes. The effects of vapors from electronic cigarettes is unclear.
- Discuss resources to stop smoking (smoking-cessation programs, medication support, self-help groups).

Carbon monoxide

- Carbon monoxide is a very dangerous gas because it binds with hemoglobin and ultimately reduces the oxygen supplied to tissues in the body.
- Carbon monoxide cannot be seen, smelled, or tasted.
- Indications of carbon monoxide poisoning include nausea, vomiting, headache, weakness, and unconsciousness.

CLIENT EDUCATION

- Ensure proper ventilation when using fuel-burning devices (lawn mowers, wood-burning and gas fireplaces, charcoal grills).
- Have gas-burning furnaces, water heaters, chimneys, flues, and appliances inspected annually.
- Flues and chimneys should be unobstructed.
- Install and maintain carbon monoxide detectors.

Food poisoning

- Most food poisoning is caused by bacteria (*Escherichia coli*, *Listeria monocytogenes*, salmonella).
- Very young, very old, pregnant, and immunocompromised individuals are at risk for complications.
- Clients who are especially at risk are instructed to follow a low-microbial diet.

Measures to prevent food poisoning
- Proper hand hygiene
- Ensuring that eggs, meat, and fish are cooked to the correct temperature
- Handling raw and cooked food separately to avoid cross-contamination
- Not using the same container, cutting board, or utensils for raw and cooked foods
- Refrigerating perishable items
- Washing raw fruits and vegetables before peeling, cutting, or eating
- Not consuming unpasteurized dairy products or untreated water

Disasters

- Natural disasters, such a tornadoes and floods, and human-made events (forest fires or explosions) can occur without warning.
- Encourage personal emergency preparedness for clients and families, which includes gathering supplies (food, water, clothing, communication devices, extra medications, and personal documents).

Ergonomic principles

Ergonomics are the factors or qualities in an object's design and/or use that contribute to comfort, safety, efficiency, and ease of use. Qs

- Body mechanics is the proper use of muscles to maintain balance, posture, and body alignment when performing a physical task. Nurses use body mechanics when providing care to clients by lifting, bending, and carrying out the activities of daily living.
- The risk of injury to the client and the nurse is reduced with the use of good body mechanics. Whenever possible, mechanical lift devices should be used to lift and transfer clients. Many health care agencies have "no manual lift" and "no solo lift" policies.
- **SEE FUNDAMENTALS CHAPTER 14: ERGONOMIC PRINCIPLES AND CLIENT POSITIONING FOR MORE INFORMATION.**

GUIDELINES TO PREVENT INJURY

- Know your agency's policies regarding lifting.
- Plan ahead for activities that require lifting, transfer, or ambulation of a client, and ask other staff members to be ready to assist at the time planned.
- Maintain good posture and exercise regularly to increase the strength of arm, leg, back, and abdominal muscles so these activities require less energy.
- Use smooth movements when lifting and moving clients to prevent injury through sudden or jerky muscle movements.
- When standing for long periods of time, flex the hip and knee through use of a foot rest. When sitting for long periods of time, keep the knees slightly higher than the hips.
- Avoid repetitive movements of the hands, wrists, and shoulders. Take a break every 15 to 20 min to flex and stretch joints and muscles.
- Maintain good posture (head and neck in straight line with pelvis) to avoid neck flexion and hunched shoulders, which can cause impingement of nerves in the neck.
- Avoid twisting the spine or bending at the waist (flexion) to minimize the risk for injury.
- Keep objects close to the body core when lifting, and bend the knees to keep the center of gravity closer to the ground.
- When lifting an object from the floor, flex the hips, knees, and back. Get the object to thigh level, keeping the knees bent and straightening the back. Stand up while holding the object as close as possible to the body, bringing the load to the center of gravity to increase stability and decrease back strain.
- Use assistive devices whenever possible, and seek assistance whenever it is needed.
- Face the direction of movement when moving a client.
- Use own body as a counterweight when pushing or pulling, which makes the movement easier.
- Sliding, rolling, and pushing require less energy than lifting and have less risk for injury.
- Avoid twisting the thoracic spine and bending the back while the hips and knees are straight.
- Assess the client's ability to help with repositioning and mobility (balance, muscle strength, endurance).
- Determine the need for additional personnel or assistive devices (transfer belt, hydraulic lift, sliding board, gait belt).

Application Exercises

1. A home health nurse is assessing the safety of a client's home. The nurse should identify which of the following factors as increasing the client's risk for falls? (Select all that apply.)

   A. History of a previous fall

   B. Reduced vision

   C. Impaired memory

   D. Takes rosuvastatin

   E. Uses a night light

   F. Kyphosis

2. A nurse on an acute care unit is caring for a client following a total hip arthroplasty. The client is confused, moving the affected leg into positions that could dislocate the new hip joint, and repeatedly attempting to get out of bed. After determining that restraint application is indicated, which of the following actions should the nurse take? (Select all that apply.)

   A. Secure the restraint to the frame of the bed.

   B. Get a prescription for restraints from the provider.

   C. Have a family member sign the consent for restraints.

   D. Tie the restraint to the side rail using a double knot.

   E. Ensure that only one finger can be inserted between the restraint and the client.

3. A nurse is observing a newly licensed nurse and an assistive personnel (AP) pull a client up in bed using a drawsheet. Which of the following actions by the newly licensed nurse indicates an understanding of this technique?

   A. The nurse stands with both feet together.

   B. The nurse uses their body weight to counter the client's weight.

   C. The nurse's feet are facing inward, toward the center of the bed.

   D. The nurse rotates the waist while pulling the client upward.

4. A nurse is planning safety interventions at a new clinic. Which of the following interventions should the nurse include?

   A. Have staff who will be performing x-rays wear dosimeters.

   B. Provide both latex and non-latex gloves for employees.

   C. Place sharps containers outside client rooms.

   D. Provide electrical tape for staff to repair frayed cords.

5. A nurse is reviewing the hospital's fire safety policies and procedures with newly hired assistive personnel. The nurse is describing what to do when there is a fire in a client's trash can. Which of the following information should the nurse include? (Select all that apply.)

   A. The first step is to pull the alarm.

   B. Use a Class C fire extinguisher to put out the fire.

   C. Instruct ambulatory clients to evacuate to a safe place.

   D. Pull the pin on the fire extinguisher prior to use.

   E. Close all doors.

Active Learning Scenario

A nurse manager is preparing to discuss electrical safety with the nurses on the unit. List the information that should be included in the discussion for each of the following aspects of safety. Use the ATI Active Learning Template: Basic Concept to complete this item.

UNDERLYING PRINCIPLES

• Identify the frequency in which the nurse should check equipment.

• List four measures to prevent electrical shock.

Application Exercises Key

1. A. **CORRECT:** A client who has had a previous fall
   is at an increased risk for another fall.
   B. **CORRECT:** Reduced vision increases the client's risk
   for tripping over equipment and furniture.
   C. **CORRECT:** A client who has impaired memory
   is at an increased risk for falls due to not asking
   for help with ambulation or ADLs.
   D. This medication does not place the client at risk for falls.
   E. The use of night lights and adequate
   lighting decreases the risk for falls.
   F. **CORRECT:** Kyphosis, which is a type of curvature of
   the spine, alters the client's posture and center of
   balance and can place the client at risk for falls.

   Ⓝ *NCLEX® Connection: Safety and Infection Control, Home Safety*

2. A. **CORRECT:** Secure the restraint to a movable
   part of the bed frame.
   B. **CORRECT:** Obtain a prescription from the provider
   as soon as possible, typically within 1 hr.
   C. **CORRECT:** Most agencies encourage informed consent
   for restraints. Instruct the family on the purpose of,
   alternatives to, and requirements for restraints.
   D. A quick-release knot must be used to secure the restraint.
   E. The distance between the restraint and the
   client should be two finger widths.

   Ⓝ *NCLEX® Connection: Safety and Infection Control, Use of
   Restraints/Safety Devices*

3. A. When pulling a client up in bed, spread both legs
   apart to create a wide base of support.
   B. **CORRECT:** Use body weight to counter the
   client's weight to make pulling easier.
   C. Both feet should point at the head of the bed
   instead of the center of the bed.
   D. Avoid rotating and twisting while moving
   clients to prevent injury.

   Ⓝ *NCLEX® Connection: Management of Care,
   Assignment, Delegation and Supervision*

4. A. **CORRECT:** Radiation is a hazardous material.
   Provide dosimeters for staff to measure their
   cumulative radiation exposure.
   B. Use non-latex products when possible, to reduce the
   risk for latex allergy development or reactions.
   C. Place sharps containers at the point of care to
   reduce the risk for needlestick injury.
   D. Instruct staff to remove equipment with frayed
   cords from the client care area, and have
   someone certified repair the equipment.

   Ⓝ *NCLEX® Connection: Safety and Infection Control, Safe Use
   of Equipment*

5. A. When a fire occurs in a client's room, the first step to take
   is to remove or evacuate the client from the room. Know
   the RACE sequence: rescue the client, pull the alarm,
   confine the fire, and then extinguish the fire.
   B. Class A fire extinguishers are used for
   paper, wood, and cloth.
   C. **CORRECT:** Ambulatory clients can walk
   by themselves to a safe place.
   D. **CORRECT:** The fire extinguisher PASS sequence is pull
   the pin, aim at the base of the fire, squeeze the lever,
   and sweep the fire extinguisher from side to side.
   E. **CORRECT:** The employee should close
   all doors to contain the fire.

   Ⓝ *NCLEX® Connection: Safety and Infection Control, Accident/
   Error/Injury Prevention*

Active Learning Scenario Key

Using the ATI Active Learning Template: Basic Concept
UNDERLYING PRINCIPLES
- The nurse should check all equipment at the
  beginning and end of each shift.
- Measures to prevent electrical shock
  ○ Ensure that all electrical equipment has a three-
    way plug and grounded outlet.
  ○ Ensure that outlet covers are used in areas
    (pediatric and mental health units).
  ○ When unplugging equipment, grasp the plug, not the cord.
  ○ Disconnect all equipment prior to cleaning.
  ○ Ensure that outlets are not overcrowded.
  ○ Use extension cords only when absolute necessary. If
    used in an open area, tape the cords to the floor.

Ⓝ *NCLEX® Connection: Safety and Infection Control, Accident/Error/
Injury Prevention*

When reviewing the following chapter, keep in mind the relevant topics and tasks of the NCLEX outline, in particular:

Safety and Infection Control

EMERGENCY RESPONSE PLAN

Use clinical decision-making/critical thinking for emergency response plan.

Determine which client(s) to recommend for discharge in a disaster situation.

REPORTING OF INCIDENT/EVENT/IRREGULAR OCCURRENCE/VARIANCE

Evaluate response to error/event/occurrence.

Identify need/situation where reporting of incident/event/ irregular occurrence/variance is appropriate.

SECURITY PLAN

Apply principles of triage and evacuation procedures/protocols.

Follow security plan and procedures (e.g., newborn nursery security, violence, controlled access).

Facility Protocols

Facility protocols refer to the plans and procedures in place to address specific issues that health care institutions face.

Nurses must understand their role in relation to development and implementation of facility protocols, including reporting incidents, disaster planning, emergency response, and security plans.

Reporting incidents

Incident reports are records of unexpected or unusual incidents that affected a client, employee, volunteer, or visitor in a health care facility.
- Facilities can also refer to incident reports as unusual occurrence or quality variance reports.
- In most states, as long as proper safeguards are employed, incident reports cannot be subpoenaed by clients or used as evidence in lawsuits.

Examples when an incident report should be filed
- Medication errors
- Procedure/treatment errors
- Equipment-related injuries/errors
- Needlestick injuries
- Client falls/injuries
- Visitor/volunteer injuries
- Threat made to client or staff
- Loss of property (dentures, jewelry, personal wheelchair)

> Nurses must ensure the safety of clients' valuables. If a client is admitted to the facility and does not have a family member present, secure the client's valuables in accordance with facility policy. If an individual requests the client's valuables, the client must identify the person and give that person permission to be in possession of the valuables.

NURSING ROLE IN REPORTING INCIDENTS

In the event of an incident that involves a client, employee, volunteer, or visitor, the nurse's priority is to assess the individual for injuries and institute any immediate care measures necessary to decrease further injury. If the incident was client-related, notify the provider and implement additional tests or treatment as prescribed. Qs

INCIDENT REPORTS
- Should be completed by the person who identifies that an unexpected event has occurred. (This might not be the individual most directly involved in the incident.)
- Should be completed as soon as possible and within 24 hr of the incident.
- Considered confidential and are not shared with the client. (Nor is it acknowledged to the client that one was completed.)
- Not placed nor mentioned in the client's health care record. However, a description of the incident should be documented factually in the client's record.
- Include an objective description of the incident and actions taken to safeguard the client, as well as assessment and treatment of any injuries sustained.
- Forwarded to the risk management department or officer (varies by facility), possibly after being reviewed by the nurse manager.
- Provide data for performance improvement studies regarding the incidence of client injuries and care-related errors. Qqi

When completing an incident report, include:
- Client's name and hospital number (or visitor's name and address if visitor injury), along with the date, time, and location of the incident
- Factual description of the incident and injuries incurred, avoiding assumptions as to the incident's cause
- Names of witnesses to the incident and client or witness comments regarding the incident
- Corrective actions that were taken, including notification of the provider and referrals
- Name and dose of any medication or identification number of any equipment involved in the incident

Disaster planning and emergency response

A **disaster** is an event that can cause serious damage, destruction, injuries, and death. In many situations, a hospital can manage the event with the support of local resources.

A **mass casualty incident (MCI)** is a catastrophic event that overwhelms local resources. Multiple resources (federal and state) are necessary to handle the crisis.

Emergency operating plan

Each facility must have an emergency operating plan (EOP). An essential component of the plan is the provision of training of all personnel regarding each component of the EOP. Nurses should understand their responsibilities in the EOP.
- Facilities accredited by the Joint Commission must have an EOP and are mandated to test the plan at least twice a year. Qs
- The EOP should interface with local, state, and federal resources.

INCIDENT REPORT

Health Care Providers

This form should not be placed in the medical record or copied

1234 Main Street
Shermer, IL 12345
1.800.555.1234

Name of person completing form: _____

Provider(s): _____

Date of incident: _____

Time of incident: _____

Date form completed: _____

Location *(select one)*

Floor/Unit: _____   Room #: _____

- ☐ Administrative Office
- ☐ Ambulatory
- ☐ Birthing Suite
- ☐ Blood Bank
- ☐ Cafeteria
- ☐ Cardiac Cath
- ☐ Central Supply
- ☐ Client's Restroom
- ☐ Client's Room
- ☐ Dialysis
- ☐ EEG
- ☐ Elevator
- ☐ Other: _____

- ☐ Emergency Department
- ☐ Extended Care Facility
- ☐ Home
- ☐ ICU
- ☐ Labor & Delivery
- ☐ Laboratory
- ☐ Lobby
- ☐ Medical Records
- ☐ Medication Room
- ☐ Mental Health
- ☐ Nuclear Medicine
- ☐ Nursery

- ☐ Nurses Station
- ☐ Obstetrics
- ☐ Operating Room
- ☐ Parking Areas
- ☐ Pathology
- ☐ Pharmacy
- ☐ Public Restroom
- ☐ Radiology
- ☐ Recovery Room
- ☐ Rehab/Therapy
- ☐ Same Day Surgery
- ☐ Stairs

Person affected by incident *(select one)*

- ☐ Employee
- ☐ Home patient
- ☐ In-patient
- ☐ Out-patient
- ☐ Provider

- ☐ Visitor
- ☐ Volunteer
- ☐ Not applicable
- ☐ Other:

List below information if not a client

Last name: _____

First name: _____

Sex: _____

Age, DOB: _____

Staff most closely involved in event *(select one)*

- ☐ Intern
- ☐ Practical Nurse
- ☐ Medical Student
- ☐ Patient Care Assistant
- ☐ Pharmacist
- ☐ Physician
- ☐ Registered Nurse
- ☐ Resident Physician

- ☐ Security
- ☐ Student Nurse
- ☐ Surgical Assistant
- ☐ Technician
- ☐ Therapist
- ☐ Volunteer
- ☐ Administrative
- ☐ Environmental

- ☐ EMS
- ☐ Physician Assistant
- ☐ Certified Registered Nurse Anesthetist
- ☐ Certified Registered Nurse Practitioner
- ☐ Not applicable
- ☐ Other: _____

Site of injury *(select one)*

- ☐ Abdomen
- ☐ Ankle(s)
- ☐ Arm(s)
- ☐ Back
- ☐ Buttocks
- ☐ Chest

- ☐ Ear(s)
- ☐ Elbow(s)
- ☐ Eye(s)
- ☐ Face
- ☐ Foot (Feet)
- ☐ Hand(s)

- ☐ Head
- ☐ Hip(s)
- ☐ Internal Injury
- ☐ Knee(s)
- ☐ Leg(s)
- ☐ Mouth

- ☐ Neck
- ☐ Nose
- ☐ Shoulder(s)
- ☐ Wrist(s)
- ☐ Not applicable
- ☐ Other: _____

Condition of the client prior to incident *(select one)*

- ☐ Agitated
- ☐ Alert
- ☐ Confused
- ☐ Disoriented

- ☐ Dizzy
- ☐ Faint
- ☐ Medicated
- ☐ Unconscious

- ☐ Uncooperative
- ☐ Weak
- ☐ Not applicable
- ☐ Other: _____

Incident report **1**

Health Care Providers INCIDENT REPORT

Description of incident (select one)

- ☐ Abrasion
- ☐ Abscess
- ☐ Amputation
- ☐ Birth injury
- ☐ Brain damage
- ☐ Burn - chemical
- ☐ Burn - electrical
- ☐ Burn - other
- ☐ Circulatory impairment
- ☐ Coma
- ☐ Concussion
- ☐ Contracture
- ☐ Contusion
- ☐ Damage to property

- ☐ Death
- ☐ Decubitus
- ☐ Dislocation
- ☐ Edema
- ☐ Foreign body
- ☐ Fracture
- ☐ Hematoma
- ☐ Hemorrhage
- ☐ Hives
- ☐ Hyperthermia
- ☐ Hypothermia
- ☐ Infection
- ☐ Inflammation
- ☐ Injury to teeth

- ☐ Laceration
- ☐ Loss of property
- ☐ Miscarriage
- ☐ Necrosis
- ☐ Obstruction
- ☐ Pain
- ☐ Paralysis
- ☐ Perforation
- ☐ Permanent disfigurement
- ☐ Poisoning
- ☐ Rape
- ☐ Rash
- ☐ Redness
- ☐ Self-inflicted injury

- ☐ Sensory impairment
- ☐ Skin puncture
- ☐ Skin tear
- ☐ Spinal damage
- ☐ Sprain
- ☐ Strain
- ☐ Suicide
- ☐ Wound disruption

- ☐ Not applicable
- ☐ Other: _____

Seen/treated by (select one)

- ☐ Attending provider
- ☐ Emergency department
- ☐ Nurse (provider notified - no prescription received)

- ☐ On-call provider
- ☐ Not applicable
- ☐ Other: _____

Treatment after incident (select one)

- ☐ Received
- ☐ Refused
- ☐ Unknown
- ☐ Not applicable

Quality information (select all that apply)

Transcription error involved?   ☐ Yes   ☐ No

Procedure
- ☐ Adverse outcome
- ☐ Application/removal of cast/sprint
- ☐ Break in sterile technique
- ☐ Client tolerance
- ☐ Client refusal
- ☐ Consent - improper
- ☐ Consent - lack of
- ☐ Delay in reporting results
- ☐ Delay in treatment
- ☐ Error in reporting result
- ☐ Other: _____

Diagnostic test
- ☐ Foreign object left in patient
- ☐ Hemorrhage
- ☐ Inappropriate operation
- ☐ Inappropriate time/sequence
- ☐ Incorrect utensil count
- ☐ Lost/mishandled specimen
- ☐ Monitoring
- ☐ Not prescribed
- ☐ Omitted
- ☐ Perforation

Treatment related
- ☐ Positioning
- ☐ Return to OR during same admission
- ☐ Surgical checklist not completed
- ☐ Transfer/moving of client
- ☐ Wrong client
- ☐ Wrong procedure
- ☐ Wrong site
- ☐ Wrong test
- ☐ Wrong treatment
- ☐ Unknown

Medication
- ☐ Break in sterile technique
- ☐ Client refusal
- ☐ Consent - improper
- ☐ Consent - lack of
- ☐ Contaminated
- ☐ Contraindicated
- ☐ Cross-match/typing error
- ☐ Delay in administration
- ☐ Discontinued by client
- ☐ Drug interaction
- ☐ Duplicated
- ☐ Food interaction
- ☐ Given after discontinued
- ☐ Given without Prescription
- ☐ Inappropriate anesthetic
- ☐ Inappropriate site

Blood
- ☐ Incomplete additives
- ☐ Incompatible blood
- ☐ Incorrect narcotic count
- ☐ Infiltration requiring treatment
- ☐ IV conscious sedation with reversal agent given
- ☐ Medication given before culture
- ☐ Mislabeled
- ☐ Out of date
- ☐ Omission
- ☐ Reaction - blood
- ☐ Reaction - correct medication
- ☐ Reaction - incorrect medication
- ☐ Repeated attempts to start IV
- ☐ Tubing not changed
- ☐ Wrong client

- ☐ Wrong Dose
- ☐ Wrong Flow Rate
- ☐ Wrong Medication (see below)
- ☐ Wrong Route
- ☐ Wrong Solution
- ☐ Wrong Time
- ☐ Other: _____

Medication:
Name:
Dosage:
Given:
Route:

Incident report   **2**

■ Health Care Providers   INCIDENT REPORT

Fall section

Surface condition (select one if applicable)
☐ Wet   ☐ Unknown
☐ Dry   ☐ Other: _____

Circumstances related to fall (select one if applicable)
☐ Ambulating - with permission   ☐ From toilet   ☐ Slipped
☐ Ambulating - without permission   ☐ From wheelchair   ☐ Tripped
☐ Dizzy   ☐ Improper footwear   ☐ Unable to follow instructions
☐ During assistance by staff   ☐ In shower   ☐ Visitor assisted client in ambulation
☐ Equipment   ☐ In tub   ☐ without staff assistance
☐ Fainted   ☐ Incontinent   ☐ Unknown
☐ Found on floor   ☐ Lost balance   ☐ Other: _____
☐ From bed   ☐ Off stretcher
☐ From chair   ☐ Off table

Client status prior to fall (complete all)
Call light on: ☐ Yes ☐ No ☐ N/A   Risk for fall assessed before incident? ☐ Yes ☐ No ☐ N/A
Restraints: ☐ Yes ☐ No ☐ N/A   Medication?   ☐ Yes ☐ No
               ☐ Refused ☐ Removed   Name: _____
Side rails: ☐ Yes ☐ No ☐ N/A   Dosage: _____
               ☐ Refused   Was restraint policy followed?   ☐ Yes ☐ No ☐ N/A
Bed position: ☐ Yes ☐ No ☐ N/A   Was client on fall precautions?   ☐ Yes ☐ No ☐ N/A

Environmental component (select one if applicable) – Equipment
☐ Disconnected   ☐ Preventive maintenance   ☐ Unknown
☐ Dislodged   ☐ Not available   ☐ Other:
☐ Equipment failure   ☐ Tampered with
☐ Equipment malfunction   ☐ User error
Device type: _____   Model #: _____   Serial #: _____

Hazardous materials and waste

☐ Spill/leak   ☐ Exposure to hazardous   ☐ Other: _____
Utilities management   material (specify): _____
☐ Medical gasses   ☐ Sewage problem   ☐ Other: _____
☐ Medical vacuum   ☐ Telephone problem
☐ Power failure   ☐ Water problem

Security

☐ Assult   ☐ Breach of confidentiality ☐ Property loss   ☐ Weapon
☐ Altercation   ☐ Gun   ☐ Property damage   ☐
☐ Other:
Miscellaneous component (select all that apply)
☐ Blood borne exposure   ☐ Provider complaint   ☐ Unknown
☐ Client/visitor/family complain ☐ Readmission in 72 hours   ☐ Other: _____
☐ Client refused treatment   ☐ Staff complaint
☐ Elopement   ☐ Unauthorized alcohol
☐ Fire   ☐ Unauthorized drugs
☐ Left AMA   ☐ Unplanned transfer to critical care
☐ Needle stick
Detailed description of the incident:
_____
_____
_____
_____
_____
_____

Incident report **3**

Internal and external emergencies

Disasters that health care facilities face include internal and external emergencies.

Internal emergencies occur within a facility and include loss of electric power or potable (drinkable) water, and severe damage or casualties related to fire, weather (tornado, hurricane), explosion, or terrorist act. Readiness includes safety and hazardous materials protocols, and infection control policies and practices.

External emergencies affect a facility indirectly and include weather (tornado, hurricane), volcanic eruptions, earthquakes, pandemic flu, chemical plant explosions, industrial accidents, building collapses, major transportation accidents, and terrorist acts (including biological and chemical warfare). Readiness includes a plan for participation in community-wide emergencies and disasters.

Disaster response agencies

Different agencies, governmental and nongovernmental, are responsible for different levels of disaster response. Agencies that have a role in disaster response include the Federal Emergency Management Agency (FEMA), CDC, U.S. Department of Homeland Security (DHS), American Red Cross, Office of Emergency Management (OEM), and the public health system.

To receive assistance with an MCI, a state must request assistance. Federal programs include the National Incident Management System, National Domestic Preparedness Organization, and Strategic National Stockpile.

NURSING ROLE IN DISASTER PLANNING AND EMERGENCY RESPONSE

EMERGENCY RESPONSE PLANS

- Health care institutions use a planning committee to develop emergency preparedness plans. The committee reviews information regarding the potential for various types of natural and human-made emergencies based on the characteristics of the community. The committee should also determine what resources are necessary to meet potential emergencies and include this information in the plan.

- The Hospital Incident Command System (HICS) for disaster management offers a clear structure for disaster management at the facility level. Ⓠᴱᴮᴾ

- Nurses and other members of the health care team should be involved in the development of an EOP for such emergencies. Criteria under which the EOP are activated should be clear. Roles for each employee should be outlined and administrative control determined. A designated area for the area command center should be established, as well as a person to serve as the incident control manager/commander.

- Key roles in the EOP include a provider to manage client numbers and resources (medical command physician), an individual to prioritize treatment (triage officer), and a media liaison (community relations/public information officer). Further information and training is available through FEMA (http://training.fema.gov).

- The nurse should create an action plan for personal family needs.

- All-hazards preparedness for human-made events includes plans for disasters of chemical, biologic, radiologic, nuclear, and explosive nature (CBRNE).

MASS CASUALTY TRIAGE Ⓠᴛᴄ

Principles of mass casualty triage should be followed in health care institutions involved in a mass casualty event.

- These differ from the principles of triage typically followed during provision of day-to-day services in an emergency or urgent care setting. **(5.2)**

- During mass casualty events, casualties are separated related to their potential for survival, and treatment is allocated accordingly. This type of triage is based on doing the greatest good for the greatest number of people.

- Nurses can find this situation very stressful because clients who are not expected to survive are cared for last.

5.2 Categories of triage during mass casualty

Emergent or immediate (CLASS I, RED TAG)	*Urgent or delayed* (CLASS II, YELLOW TAG)	*Nonurgent or minimal* (CLASS III, GREEN TAG)	*Expectant* (CLASS IV, BLACK TAG)
Highest priority is given to clients who have life-threatening injuries but also have a high possibility of survival once they are stabilized.	Second-highest priority is given to clients who have major injuries that are not yet life-threatening and usually require treatment in 30 min to 2 hr.	The next highest priority is given to clients who have minor injuries that are not life-threatening and can wait hours to days for treatment.	The lowest priority is given to clients who are not expected to live and will be allowed to die naturally. Comfort measures can be provided, but restorative care will not.

DISCHARGE/RELOCATION OF CLIENTS

During an emergency (a fire or a mass casualty event), nurses help make decisions regarding discharging clients or relocating them so their beds can be used for clients who have higher priority needs.

Nurses can use the following criteria when identifying which clients are stable enough to discharge.

- First, discharge or relocate ambulatory clients requiring minimal care.
- Next, make arrangements for continuation of care for clients who require some assistance, which could be provided in the home or tertiary care facility.
- Do not discharge or relocate clients who are unstable or require continuing nursing care and assessment unless they are in imminent danger.

TYPES OF EMERGENCIES

Biological incidents

- Be alert to indications of a possible bioterrorism attack because early detection and management is key. Often, the manifestations are similar to other illnesses. (5.3)
- Be alert for the appearance of a disease that does not normally occur at a specific time or place, has atypical manifestations, or occurs in a specific community or people group.
- In most instances, infection from biological agents is not spread from one client to another. Management of the incident includes recognition of the occurrence, directing personnel in the proper use of personal protective equipment, and, in some situations, decontamination and isolation.
- Use appropriate isolation measures.
- Transport or move clients only if needed for treatment and care.
- Take measures to protect self and others.
- Recognize indications of infection/poisoning and identify appropriate treatment interventions.

5.3 Biological incidents and their treatment and prevention

Inhalational anthrax
MANIFESTATIONS
- Fever
- Cough
- Shortness of breath
- Muscle aches
- Mild chest pain
- Meningitis
- Shock
- Prevention: Anthrax vaccine for high-risk; ciprofloxacin & doxycycline IV/PO following exposure
- Treatment: Includes one or two additional antibiotics (vancomycin, penicillin, and anthrax antitoxin)

Cutaneous anthrax
MANIFESTATIONS
- Starts as a lesion that can be itchy
- Develops into a vesicular lesion that later becomes necrotic with the formation of black eschar
- Fever, chills

PREVENTION: Anthrax vaccine for high-risk

TREATMENT: Ciprofloxacin, doxycycline

Botulism
MANIFESTATIONS
- Difficulty swallowing
- Double vision
- Slurred speech
- Descending progressive weakness
- Nausea, vomiting, abdominal cramps
- Difficulty breathing

PREVENTION/TREATMENT
- Airway management
- Antitoxin
- Elimination of toxin

Viral hemorrhagic fevers
Examples: Ebola, yellow fever

MANIFESTATIONS
- Sore throat
- Headache
- High temperature
- Nausea, vomiting, diarrhea
- Internal and external bleeding
- Shock

PREVENTION: Vaccination available for yellow fever, Argentine hemorrhagic fever; barrier protection from infected person, isolation precautions specific to disease

TREATMENT: No cure, supportive care only; minimize invasive procedures

Plague
MANIFESTATIONS
- Forms can occur separately or in combination
- Pneumonic: fever, headache, weakness, pneumonia with shortness of breath, chest pain, cough, bloody or watery sputum
- Bubonic: swollen, tender lymph glands, fever, headache, chills, weakness
- Septicemic: fever, chills, prostration, abdominal pain, shock, disseminated intravascular coagulation, gangrene of nose and digits

PREVENTION: Contact precautions until decontaminated; droplet precautions until 72 hr after antibiotics

TREATMENT: Streptomycin/gentamicin or tetracycline/doxycycline

Smallpox
MANIFESTATIONS
- High fever
- Fatigue
- Severe headache
- Rash
- Chills
- Vomiting
- Delirium

PREVENTION: vaccine; can vaccinate within 3 days of exposure; contact and airborne precautions

TREATMENT: supportive care (prevent dehydration, provide skin care, medications for pain and fever); antibiotics for secondary infections

Tularemia
MANIFESTATIONS
- Sudden fever, chills, headache, diarrhea, muscle aches, joint pain, dry cough, progressive weakness
- If airborne, life-threatening pneumonia and systemic infection

PREVENTION: Vaccine under review by the FDA

TREATMENT: Streptomycin or gentamicin are drugs of choice; in mass causality, use doxycycline or ciprofloxacin

Chemical incidents

- Can occur as result of an accident or due to a purposeful action (terrorism).
- Take measures to protect self and avoid contact.
- Assess and intervene to maintain airway, breathing, and circulation. Administer first aid as needed.
- Remove the offending chemical by undressing the client and removing all identifiable particulate matter. Provide immediate and prolonged irrigations of contaminated areas. Irrigate skin with running water, except for dry chemicals (lye or white phosphorus). In the case of exposure to a dry chemical, brush the agent off of clothing and skin.
- Gather a specific history of the injury, if possible (name and concentration of the chemical, duration of exposure).
- Know which facilities are open to exposed clients and which are open only to unexposed clients.
- Follow the facility's emergency response plans (personal protection measures, handling and disposal of wastes, use of space and equipment, reporting).

Hazardous material incidents

- Take measures to protect self and avoid contact.
- Approach the scene with caution.
- Identify the hazardous material with available resources (emergency response guidebook, poison control centers).
- Know the location of the Safety Data Sheet (SDS) manual.
- Try to contain the material in one place prior to the arrival of the hazardous materials team.
- Decontaminate affected individuals as much as possible at or as close as possible to the scene.
  - Don gloves, gown, mask, and shoe covers to protect self from contamination.
  - Carefully and slowly remove contaminated clothing so that deposited material does not become airborne.
  - With few exceptions, water is the universal antidote. For biological hazardous materials, wash skin with copious amounts of water and antibacterial soap.
  - Place contaminated materials into large plastic bags and seal them.

Nuclear incidents

- Damage can occur from radiation, radioactive fallout, or from the force of the blast.
- Decontamination is required.
- Treatment is symptomatic for burns and puncture injuries. Some clients can remain contaminated for years.

Explosive incidents

- Most common method used for terrorist activity. Injury from the heat (decomposition), airborne metal or fragments, and temperature changes.
- Treatment depends on injury type, with burns being the most common.

Radiological incidents

- Amount of exposure is related to duration of exposure, distance from source, and amount of shielding.
- The facility where victims are treated should activate interventions to prevent contamination of treatment areas (floors, furniture, air vents, and ducts should be covered; radiation-contaminated waste should be disposed of according to procedural guidelines).
- Wear water-resistant gowns, double-glove, and fully cover bodies with caps, booties, masks, and goggles.
- Wear radiation or dosimetry badges to monitor the amount of radiation exposure.
- Survey clients initially with a radiation meter to determine the amount of contamination.
- Decontamination with soap and water and disposable towels should occur prior to the client entering the facility. Water runoff will be contaminated and should be contained.
- After decontamination, resurvey clients for residual contamination, and continue irrigation of the skin until the client is free of all contamination.

Security plans

- All facilities should have security plans in place that include preventive, protective, and response measures designed for identified security needs.
- Security issues faced by health care facilities include admission of potentially dangerous individuals, vandalism, infant abduction, and information theft.
- The International Association for Healthcare Security & Safety (IAHSS) provides recommendations for the development of security plans.

NURSING ROLE IN SECURITY PLANS

Nurses should be prepared to take immediate action when breaches in security occur. Time is of the essence in preventing a breach in security. Qs

SECURITY MEASURES

- An identification system that identifies employees, volunteers, physicians, students, and regularly scheduled contract services staff as authorized personnel of the facility
- Electronic security systems in high-risk areas (the maternal newborn unit to prevent infant abductions, the emergency department to prevent unauthorized entrance)
  - Key code access into and out of high-risk areas
  - Wrist bands that electronically link parents and their infant
  - Alarms integrated with closed-circuit television cameras

Emergency designations

Health care facilities have color code designations for emergencies. These vary between institutions, but some examples are:
- Code Red: fire
- Code Pink: newborn/infant/child abduction
- Code Orange: chemical spill
- Code Blue: medical emergency
- Code Gray: tornado
- Code Black: bomb threat

In addition, some hospitals use plain language descriptions for significant alerts (violent situations or evacuations [example "Facility Alert: active shooter, main lobby."]).

Nurses should be familiar with procedures and policies that outline proper measures to take when one of these emergencies are called.

Fire

In the event of a fire or suspected threat, follow the RACE mnemonic to guide the order of actions, and the PASS mnemonic for use of a fire extinguisher, if indicated.
(**SEE CHAPTER 4: MAINTAINING A SAFE ENVIRONMENT.**)
- In most facilities, when the fire alarm system is activated, some systems are automatically shut down (the oxygen flow system).
- Ensure fire doors are not blocked; many will close automatically when the alarm system is activated.

Severe thunderstorm/tornado

- Draw shades, and close drapes to protect against shattering glass.
- Lower all beds to the lowest position, and move beds away from the windows.
- Place blankets over all clients who are confined to beds.
- Close all doors.
- Relocate ambulatory clients into the hallways (away from windows) or other secure location designated by the facility.
- Do not use elevators.
- Turn on the severe weather channel to monitor severe weather warnings.

Bomb threat

- If a bomb-like device is located, do not touch it. Clear the area, and isolate the device as much as possible by closing doors, for example.
- Notify the appropriate authorities and personnel (police, administrator, director of nursing).
- Cooperate with police and others: Assist to conduct search as needed, provide copies of floor plans, have master keys available, and watch for and isolate suspicious objects (packages and boxes).
- Keep elevators available for authorities.
- Remain calm and alert, and try not to alarm clients.

When a phone call is received
- Extend the conversation as long as possible.
- Listen for distinguishing background noises (music, voices, traffic, airplanes).
- Note distinguishing voice characteristics of the caller.
- Ask where and when the bomb is set to explode.
- Note whether the caller is familiar with the physical arrangement of the facility.

Active shooter situation

These situations involve one or more persons trying to kill people in a confined area. Recommendations from the U.S. Department of Homeland Security on responding to an active shooter situation involve running, hiding, and fighting.
- **Running** involves evacuation if there is a clear path of exit. This includes leaving without belongings and instructing others to follow but not waiting if they do not. It also includes keeping others from entering an area where the shooter might be.
- **Hiding** is the second option if it is not possible to evacuate the area. Key concepts include hiding out of view, locking or blocking the entry to the location, and remaining quiet and preventing noises (cell phones).
- **Fighting** involves taking action against the shooter if evacuating and hiding are not options. This should be done only if danger is imminent. This involves aggressive acts to stop or wound the shooter by throwing items or using weapons and yelling.
- General measures include calling 911 when safe, even if unable to talk; not attempting to move wounded people until the scene is safe; and remaining calm and quiet. If police enter the scene, keep hands visible and remain cooperative.

1. A nurse discovers that a client was administered an antihypertensive medication in error. Identify the appropriate sequence of steps that the nurse should take using the following actions.

   A. Call the provider.

   B. Check vital signs.

   C. Notify the risk manager.

   D. Complete an incident report.

   E. Instruct the client to remain in bed until further notice.

2. A nurse manager is explaining the use of incident reports to a group of nurses in an orientation program. Which of the following information should the nurse manager include? (Select all that apply.)

   A. A description of the incident should be documented in the client's health care record.

   B. The client should sign as a witness on the incident report.

   C. Incident reports include a description of the incident and actions taken.

   D. A copy of the incident report should be placed in the client's health care record.

   E. The risk management department investigates the incident.

3. A nurse is discussing disaster planning with the board members of a hospital. Which of the following individuals should the nurse expect to request extra supplies and staffing for the facility?

   A. Incident commander

   B. Medical command physician

   C. Triage officer

   D. Media liaison

4. A community experiences an outbreak of meningitis, and hospital beds are urgently needed. Which of the following clients should the nurse recommend for discharge?

   A. A client newly admitted with angina and a history of myocardial infarction 1 year ago

   B. A client who was preadmitted for rotator cuff surgery and has diabetes mellitus type 2

   C. A client admitted the day before with pneumonia and dehydration

   D. A client who has a fractured hip and is scheduled for total hip replacement the next day

5. A nurse on a sixth-floor medical-surgical unit is advised that a severe weather alert code has been activated. Which of the following actions should the nurse take? (Select all that apply.)

   A. Open window shades or drapes to provide better visibility of the external environment.

   B. Move beds of nonambulatory clients away from windows.

   C. Relocate ambulatory clients into the hallways.

   D. Use the elevators to move clients to lower levels.

   E. Turn the radio on for severe weather warnings.

Active Learning Scenario

A nurse serving on a disaster preparedness committee is reviewing information about smallpox. Use the ATI Active Learning Template: System Disorder to complete this item.

EXPECTED FINDINGS: List at least three manifestations.

NURSING CARE: List at least two treatment measures.

1. *Correct order*
   B. The first action to take using the nursing process is to check the client for hypotension by measuring vital signs.
   E. Next, instruct the client to remain in bed to prevent a fall due to the risk of hypotension.
   A. Then notify the provider, who can prescribe a medication to treat hypotension.
   D. Next, complete an incident report that is thorough, objective, and accurate.
   C. The last step to take is to report the incident to the risk manager.

   Ⓝ *NCLEX® Connection: Safety and Infection Control, Reporting of Incident/Event/Irregular Occurrence Variance*

2. A. **CORRECT:** Document a factual description of the event in the client's health care record.
   B. Do not inform the client or individual involved that an incident report has been filed. Incident reports are for facility quality assurance.
   C. **CORRECT:** In addition to providing an accurate description of the event, also document the actions taken following the event.
   D. Do not place the incident report in the client's health care record in order to shield it from discovery in the event of a lawsuit.
   E. **CORRECT:** Expect a risk manager to investigate all incidents as part of the agency's quality assurance program.

   Ⓝ *NCLEX® Connection: Safety and Infection Control, Reporting of Incident/Event/Irregular Occurrence Variance*

3. A. Expect the incident commander to manage the incident and key leaders within the facility.
   B. **CORRECT:** Expect the medical command physician to oversee use of resources (equipment and personnel).
   C. Expect the triage officer to prioritize the treatment of incoming clients.
   D. Expect the media liaison to communicate with members of the media and press on behalf of the facility.

   Ⓝ *NCLEX® Connection: Safety and Infection Control, Emergency Response Plan*

4. A. Recognize that a client who has angina is at risk for a cardiac event. Do not recommend this client for discharge because the client is unstable.
   B. **CORRECT:** Identify that this client is stable and their condition can be managed at home with surgery rescheduled. This meets the criteria of first discharging clients who are ambulatory and require minimal care.
   C. Recognize that a client who has dehydration and active infection requires ongoing nursing care. Do not recommend this client for discharge because the client is unstable.
   D. Recognize that a client who has hip fracture is unstable and at risk for further damage to the hip. If the client were 1 day or more postoperative, discharging the client to a tertiary facility might have been possible.

   Ⓝ *NCLEX® Connection: Safety and Infection Control, Emergency Response Plan*

5. A. Close the window shades and drapes to protect clients from shattering glass.
   B. **CORRECT:** Move the beds of nonambulatory clients away from windows to protect clients from shattering glass.
   C. **CORRECT:** Relocate ambulatory clients into the hallway to protect the clients from shattering glass.
   D. Instruct others that it is unsafe to use the elevator.
   E. **CORRECT:** Use the radio to monitor the activity of the storm.

   Ⓝ *NCLEX® Connection: Safety and Infection Control, Emergency Response Plan*

Using the ATI Active Learning Template: System Disorder

EXPECTED FINDINGS
- High fever
- Fatigue
- Severe headache
- Rash
- Chills
- Vomiting
- Delirium

NURSING CARE
- Prevent dehydration.
- Provide skin care.
- Administer medications for pain and fever.
- Provide vaccination if within 3 days of exposure.
- Implement contact and airborne precautions.
- Administer antibiotics for secondary infections.

Ⓝ *NCLEX® Connection: Safety and Infection Control, Emergency Response Plan*

References

American Nurses Credentialing Center (2018). Redesignation for Magnet® facilities. Retrieved from https://www.nursingworld. org/organizational-programs/magnet/redesignation/

Berman, A., Snyder, S., & Frandsen, G. (2016). *Kozier & Erb's fundamentals of nursing: Concepts, process, and practice* (10th ed.). Upper Saddle River, NJ: Prentice-Hall.

Centers for Disease Control and Prevention (2014). During a tornado. Retrieved from https://www.cdc.gov/disasters/tornadoes/during.html

Centers for Disease Control and Prevention (2017). Smallpox. Retrieved from https://www.cdc.gov/smallpox

Cherry, B., & Jacob, S. R. (2017). *Contemporary nursing: Issues, trends, & management* (7th ed.). St. Louis, MO: Elsevier.

Federal Emergency Management Agency. (2018). Welcome to national preparedness. Retrieved from http://training.fema.gov

Ignatavicius, D. D., Workman, M. L., & Rebar, C. R. (2018). *Medical-Surgical nursing: Concepts for Interprofessional collaborative care* (9th ed.). St. Louis, MO.

Marquis, B. L., & Huston, C. J. (2017). *Leadership roles and management functions in nursing: Theory and application* (9th ed.). Philadelphia: Wolters Kluwer.

National Council of State Boards of Nursing. (2013). Outline of NCSBN's transition to practice (TTP) modules. Retrieved from https://www.ncsbn.org/2013_TransitiontoPractice_Modules.pdf

Pagana, K. D., & Pagana, T. J. (2018). *Mosby's manual of diagnostic and laboratory tests* (6th ed.). St. Louis: Elsevier.

Potter, P. A., Perry, A. G., Stockert, P., & Hall, A. (2017). *Fundamentals of nursing* (9th ed.). St. Louis, MO: Elsevier.

Weiss, S. A., & Tappen, R. M. (2015). *Essentials of nursing leadership & management* (6th ed.). Philadelphia: F.A. Davis Company.

STUDENT NAME _____

CONCEPT_____ REVIEW MODULE CHAPTER_____

Related Content
(E.G., DELEGATION, LEVELS OF PREVENTION, ADVANCE DIRECTIVES)

Underlying Principles

Nursing Interventions
WHO? WHEN? WHY? HOW?

STUDENT NAME _____

PROCEDURE NAME _____ _____ REVIEW MODULE CHAPTER_____

Description of Procedure

Indications

Interpretation of Findings

Potential Complications

CONSIDERATIONS

Nursing Interventions (pre, intra, post)

Client Education

Nursing Interventions

Growth and Development

STUDENT NAME _____

DEVELOPMENTAL STAGE _____ REVIEW MODULE CHAPTER_____

EXPECTED GROWTH AND DEVELOPMENT

Physical Development	Cognitive Development	Psychosocial Development	Age-Appropriate Activities

Health Promotion

Immunizations	Health Screening	Nutrition	Injury Prevention

STUDENT NAME _____

MEDICATION _____ REVIEW MODULE CHAPTER_____

CATEGORY CLASS_____

PURPOSE OF MEDICATION

Expected Pharmacological Action

Therapeutic Use

Complications

Medication Administration

Contraindications/Precautions

Nursing Interventions

Interactions

Client Education

Evaluation of Medication Effectiveness

STUDENT NAME _____

SKILL NAME_____ REVIEW MODULE CHAPTER_____

Description of Skill

Indications

CONSIDERATIONS

Nursing Interventions (pre, intra, post)

Outcomes/Evaluation

Client Education

Potential Complications

Nursing Interventions

System Disorder

STUDENT NAME _____

DISORDER/DISEASE PROCESS _____ REVIEW MODULE CHAPTER_____

Alterations in Health (Diagnosis)	Pathophysiology Related to Client Problem	Health Promotion and Disease Prevention

ASSESSMENT

Risk Factors	Expected Findings

Laboratory Tests	Diagnostic Procedures

SAFETY CONSIDERATIONS

PATIENT-CENTERED CARE

Nursing Care	Medications	Client Education

Therapeutic Procedures		Interprofessional Care

Complications

ACTIVE LEARNING TEMPLATE: *Therapeutic Procedure*

STUDENT NAME _____

PROCEDURE NAME _____ REVIEW MODULE CHAPTER_____

Description of Procedure

Indications

Outcomes/Evaluation

Potential Complications

CONSIDERATIONS

Nursing Interventions (pre, intra, post)

Client Education

Nursing Interventions

Concept Analysis

STUDENT NAME _____

CONCEPT ANALYSIS_____

Defining Characteristics

Antecedents

(WHAT MUST OCCUR/BE IN PLACE FOR
CONCEPT TO EXIST/FUNCTION PROPERLY)

Negative Consequences

(RESULTS FROM IMPAIRED ANTECEDENT —
COMPLETE WITH FACULTY ASSISTANCE)

Related Concepts

(REVIEW LIST OF CONCEPTS AND IDENTIFY, WHICH
CAN BE AFFECTED BY THE STATUS OF THIS CONCEPT
— COMPLETE WITH FACULTY ASSISTANCE)

Exemplars